THRIVE TO 95 AND BEYOND

Taking Control of your Aging Journey

ELIZABETH PHINNEY

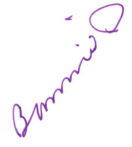

BALBOA.PRESS
A DIVISION OF HAY HOUSE

Copyright © 2023 Elizabeth Phinney.

All rights reserved. No part of this book may be used or reproduced by any means, graphic, electronic, or mechanical, including photocopying, recording, taping or by any information storage retrieval system without the written permission of the author except in the case of brief quotations embodied in critical articles and reviews.

Balboa Press books may be ordered through booksellers or by contacting:

Balboa Press
A Division of Hay House
1663 Liberty Drive
Bloomington, IN 47403
www.balboapress.com
844-682-1282

Because of the dynamic nature of the Internet, any web addresses or links contained in this book may have changed since publication and may no longer be valid. The views expressed in this work are solely those of the author and do not necessarily reflect the views of the publisher, and the publisher hereby disclaims any responsibility for them.

The author of this book does not dispense medical advice or prescribe the use of any technique as a form of treatment for physical, emotional, or medical problems without the advice of a physician, either directly or indirectly. The intent of the author is only to offer information of a general nature to help you in your quest for physical, emotional and spiritual well-being. In the event you use any of the information in this book for yourself, which is your constitutional right, the author and the publisher assume no responsibility for your actions.

Printed in the United States of America

ISBN: 979-8-7652-3631-4 (sc)
ISBN: 979-8-7652-3633-8 (hc)
ISBN: 979-8-7652-3632-1 (e)

Library of Congress Control Number: 2022920993

Balboa Press rev. date: 06/09/2023

INTRODUCTION

The following story illustrates why you need to read this book.

In celebration of my 70th birthday, I decided to take three months off at the beginning of 2023. Some very generous friends allowed me to crash at their places from Florida to Arizona to California. As I did most days, while with my friend in California, I took an afternoon walk. When I was almost back to her place, I fell. Somehow, I just fell – tripped over my own feet. I truly have no idea what triggered the fall. But it was bad – I mean, really bad.

Knowing as much as I do about human physiology, muscles and joints, I knew I was in serious trouble. I figured I probably had a hairline fracture of my right ankle as well as tissue damage surrounding the ankle bone. My left groin was the most painful spot so I knew there were significant tissue tears there – from the top of my inner thigh down about 6 or 7 inches. Then there was the area from my left armpit down my left side into my left breast. I was in pain. Needless to say, I immediately started icing all the injured places and resting to help the healing process.

I could barely walk; every step was extremely uncomfortable. Getting up and down from a chair was tough because I couldn't lean on my left side to help hoist myself up. Adjusting positions in bed was incredibly painful. I was a mess.

And I was scared. I knew the fracture would take a couple of months to heal, but complete healing of the tissue damage, especially at 70 years old, can take over a year. I was planning to make exercise videos and begin promoting this book upon my return home. How on earth was I going to do all that with these injuries?

Needless to say, I did not exercise for the rest of my trip. As the injuries slowly began to get better, I was able to do more things without pain. On the way home, I visited my daughter and her boyfriend in Washington, D.C. It was exactly one month after my fall. I wanted to see the cherry blossoms, and we ended up taking about a 5-mile walk around the city. I was pain-free, both during and after the walk! In other words, I was completely healed, in one month! And let me repeat, I am 70 years old. A miracle? Actually, no. It's a message. A message I needed to bring to this book and to you.

I am in very good shape. Because I strength train and stretch on a regular basis and eat a very nutritious diet, my body was able to heal very quickly. If I were not as strong and flexible and healthy as I am, I guarantee I would have been in healing mode for many long months.

I wanted to share this story of my quick recovery to help you understand how important strengthening and stretching are for your body and your well-being. The bottom line is that you can recover just as quickly as I did from a fall if you make the right choices for your body and follow the guidelines set forth within these pages. I encourage you to do so. The confidence I have gained since that fall is amazing – it is proof positive that my regimen works, even better than I knew!

I first had the notion of writing a book about ten years ago, after I had been a personal trainer for twelve years. By then I had worked with hundreds of people, mainly women, and had discovered that too often people would find themselves turning 70 or 80 and be disillusioned with how their health had declined. In the worst cases, some debilitating disease had taken hold.

They felt helpless in the face of the aging trauma that was slowly happening to them. Some figured they were just getting older and it was just their time. But others were truly at a loss. They thought they had been doing all the right things to maintain good health, and yet their bodies were failing them. (In every single instance, each person had their own perspective of what those "right things" were.)

Universally, people were the "victims" of whatever response to aging they had. No one was able to recognize the control they had over how their bodies would age.

With this book I hope to make the point that we can each be our own best advocate for aging the way we want to age. You do need to keep in mind that up to now, your body has already been storing up certain reactions based on your behavior over the years. Ideally, from this moment forward, you will be able to be more assertive in your healthy behavior and recognize the gifts you can give to your body that are, in fact, within your control.

Much of what you will be reading you may have heard before. However, I do not believe you have ever heard it presented in the way it is presented here. This is not so much a "how to" book as it is a "why not" or a "what if" book. The choice is always up to you.

The behaviors you choose now will affect where you will be physiologically 20 years from now – maybe sooner, maybe later. And make no mistake – this long-term planning is not hardwired into our DNA. It will take time to rewire your brain to create new habits and new muscle memory so that your new behaviors become second nature.

The question, then, is whether you will begin your lifestyle transition now, when you can slowly but surely make the necessary changes over a period of years, or wait until you have been diagnosed with cancer or heart disease or some auto-immune disorder, when your efforts would have to be directed toward reversing the progress of a disease rather than preventing it from happening in the first place.

My mission in writing this book is to help people take control of their physical future. Many books have been published on the subject. This book, obviously, represents my opinions, the way I view things, what I personally practice and what I have shared thousands of times with my clients. I am neither a scientist nor a doctor. Whatever scientific or medical information you find within these pages that interests you, I strongly suggest that you take the idea and explore it further on your own. There is so much information out there – good and bad – and I believe it is very important that we, as individuals, do our own research so we can learn and practice what it is that inspires us and teaches us to be better and healthier people. It must be stated that whatever activities or practices you adopt from information you have read within this book, you do so at your own risk.

For those of you who have already started "doing the right thing," I hope this book brings you more ideas to keep your journey as fulfilling as possible. For those of you who didn't realize that now is the time, I hope you find these ideas inspiring, giving you the push you need to get this ball rolling. And for those of you who truly had no idea that you had any power over how you age, I hope you learn and adopt these practices so that you are able to continue to fulfill your dreams and desires well into your 90s … so that you can truly *Thrive to 95 and Beyond*.

THIS IS NO ORDINARY DEDICATION

The dedication of this book requires a bit of a backstory.

It wasn't until 2012 that I realized that I should write a book. I had been attending a lot of conferences and I went to one about that subject. From there, I contributed to an anthology called **The Expert Success Solution**. It was a fabulous collaboration of 22 people, each with our own specialty and vision for success. It became a #1 International Best Seller on Amazon, which allows me the "Best Selling Author" title. That book was published in 2014 and I now "had the bug" to write my own book.

I truly had no idea what that would entail – certainly I knew how to write, but was completely naïve as to the dedication and diligence the task would require. Finally, in November of 2016, I purchased the Hay House Writers Workshop. With the purchase of the course came the possibility that my manuscript would be published by Hay House – they would pick one from all the attendees. That got me to compile chapters and an outline of each chapter and helped me to sort out exactly what I wanted to write about. My dear friend and coach Dianne helped me do the whole thing and it was submitted in February 2017. My book was not chosen, but the hard part was done…or so I thought.

Now, there was a parallel story going on simultaneously over these years in which I am procrastinating about writing this book. There is no easy way to introduce this story: My son, Blake, was killed by a hit-and-run driver in September of 2009, three weeks after his 21st birthday. I had no idea that this lifetime would challenge me this way nor did I ever imagine I would need this level of strength to live. Fortunately, I am a strong believer in the afterlife and communications from the other side. One year after his death, my son spoke to me over my right shoulder, "Mom, you've had your year. It is time to get back out there and do your thing." That was it.

I began a 3-year quest to learn what I needed to know to fulfill my destiny. I listened to seminars and webinars and found gurus and teachers who were doing exactly what I wanted to be doing – speaking to an audience. I needed to learn how to spread the word in the 2000s, so I learned how to do social media, public relations and marketing.

I met amazing people from all over the country and the world. Many of them have been incredibly supportive in helping to get this book written.

When I got home, I began to attend local events, averaging 8-9 each month. Alas, none of this got me any closer to writing the book.

Finally, about a year after the Hay House submission, my son, who was never shy with his opinions nor with his delivery of them, returned with a message, again over the right shoulder. "Just write the f***ing book, Mom. Just write the f***ing book!" And that was it. That's all I needed to hear. I got to work. Little did I know that it would still take me another 4 years to complete this intense labor of love, but so it has. On occasion, I would hear his charming message in my right ear whenever I was not being as diligent as I could be. He has been very patient.

The real push, the final push, came in February 2022. I responded to a new member of the BodSpir® Membership Program with a simple welcome email. This was her reply:

Hi Elizabeth!

I found you through a very persistent butterfly. A few months ago, I was out for a walk with one of the children I nanny. Ever since I turned 50, I have been having issues with stamina and knew I needed to find a proper exercise program. During that walk, a monarch butterfly was very present and persistent in making sure that I not only acknowledged its presence but spoke to it out loud. So, the 3-year-old I was with and I started to talk to the butterfly. We told it how beautiful it was and how grateful we were to see it. It followed us all the way home. Once in the driveway, the butterfly flew to the back of my car and landed on the dealership sticker on my trunk - Blake Motors. It was then that I realized and said, "Blake!! Is that you?" It was then that it flew right to me and landed on my right shoulder. Boy oh boy, was that a happy cry.

That night I was in front of my computer. I logged onto YouTube and what do I see but a thumbnail for a "Fitness After 45" chat with Elizabeth Phinney. So here I am. Sent by Blake.

I have collected my accessories that were suggested by you and now I begin this journey.

I hope you and all you love are well!

Best wishes,
Sandi (First Nanny to Blake)

Her response completely astounded me. I had not been in touch with Sandi since she stopped being Blake's nanny when he was still a small baby and that was 33+ years before. I wrote her back immediately:

Needless to say, I am in a bit of shock after reading your email.

Not just from all the synchronicities leading you to me, but also in the fact that Blake comes to me as a monarch butterfly!!

He is remarkable and tenacious, for sure!

We set up a Zoom call for later in the week. In firming that up, I said:

I will send you the link right before 7:00pm on Thursday! Will be fascinating, as our conversation evolves, to learn why Blake wanted to get us together!

See you soon!

But it was her reply that took everything way beyond synchronicity to actual proof that she was truly in communication with him:

I agree! However, I do think it has something to do with a book that needs to be written.

A BOOK THAT NEEDS TO BE WRITTEN?? Was she kidding? Had he really gone that far to find her to make sure that I would "just write the f***ing book!"?

Needless to say, once I learned the extent to which Blake had gone to get me to finish the book, I got right to it and found the discipline I needed to complete the project, my labor of love!!

I later learned that the day Sandi first came across the butterfly was August 28, Blake's birthday.

So, dear Sandi, I thank you so much for your recent return to my life and the endless gifts you have given me in my communications and connection with Blake. *Your* presence has enlivened *his* presence in my life every day. I can't thank you enough for my revitalized awakening and your on-going care and friendship.

It is to my dear son, Blake, that this book is dedicated. His death gave me a strength of character that I never knew existed inside of me. And his persistent support and determination to get his mother to write this book shows a love so powerful, it literally crossed dimensions.

And, to you, dear reader, I wish you the strength and determination you will need to take control of how you age for the rest of your life.

TABLE OF CONTENTS

Chapter 1:	Oh, My Aging Body!	1
Chapter 2:	Exercise is a Gift	23
Chapter 3:	Excuses, Excuses	37
Chapter 4:	Motivation vs. Inspiration	57
Chapter 5:	Bodspir® Meditative Strength Training™ the Unique Technique	71
Chapter 6:	Breathing: It's Not Just for Oxygen Anymore	87
Chapter 7:	Flexibility is the Key to Mobility	97
Chapter 8:	The Forgotten Muscle	113
Chapter 9:	You are What You Eat – Literally!	125
Chapter 10:	The Mind-Body Partnership	159
Chapter 11:	I. A.M. H.E.R.E. The Seven Steps to Controlling Your Physical Future	177
Chapter 12:	Stress – The Silent Saboteur	207
Chapter 13:	Your ~~Fiscal~~ Physical Retirement Plan	223
Chapter 14:	Mobility for Life: Emotions, Attitudes, and the Ultimate Gift	259

Chapter 1

OH, MY AGING BODY!

"It's not how old you are, it's how you are old."

Jules Renard

It can start anywhere or anytime.

You can be as young as thirty-five, or as old as seventy-five, but it *will* happen. It is inevitable and it is our destiny.

In the blink of an eye, we see the first sign of aging! We might shrug it off and not relate the issue to aging. We might keep a watchful eye on it, admitting to ourselves something is going on, but tell ourselves it is nothing to be concerned about right now.

Or it might stop us dead in our tracks, and we find ourselves doing a silent scream, something like, "OMG!!! When did I get old?"

The truth is, aging begins a lot sooner than we think. It actually begins as soon as we stop growing, somewhere between years 20 and 24. But, the signs of aging don't start to appear until much later. A good 20 to 30 years later!

THE FOUR KINDS OF AGING

There are four different kinds of aging that are considered influential, affecting our mindset, lifestyle and activities.

The Chronological Age

The actual number of years you have lived, from your birth day to the current day.

The Psychological Age

The age you mentally believe yourself to be. This can run the gamut. There are the people who think they are much younger than they are, and there are others who think they are much older. What is important to remember with psychological aging is that you are exactly what you *think* you are. So, if you are 72 years old and you think 72 is old, then, you will, in fact, be old at 72. Likewise, if you are 72 years old and you think 72 is young, you will feel much younger. Your thoughts will determine how youthful or old you are.

The Social/Cultural Age

The attitude of those around you in judging your chronological age, as well as the culture of the area you live in, play a large role and can dictate the quality of your life, whatever your age is. In some cultures, such as Abkhazia in Georgia, formerly of Russia, people are living up to 110 years or more. And they are active: riding horses and swimming in ice cold streams.[1] Because the life expectancy is so long and there are so many people living past 100 years, the quality of life and attitude towards 80- and 90-year-olds and centenarians is much different. Because the culture has these people conceptually younger and more vibrant, the people act younger and more vibrant. The culture of the area dictates the quality of the life.

---

[1] Living Beyond Miracles, Dr. Deepak Chopra with Dr. Wayne Dyer

The Biological Age

Biological age is the physiological age describing how well or poorly your body is functioning relative to your chronological age. Like the psychological age, this also runs the gamut and has a direct correlation to what we think and believe. When we think we are old, our bodies tend to react that way. The power of our mind can have a dramatic effect on our physiological age. Instead of focusing on how old you are chronologically, focus on how young you feel.

Another more serious factor with biological aging relates to having been through a severe illness. When we have no choice but to spend a significant and crucial length of time healing from a serious illness, our bodies will biologically age. When we are well again and can change our behavior, doing what we need to do to stay healthy, we can reverse much of the aging that has taken place.

What is interesting about these aging categories is only one of them is certain, steadfast and cannot be changed. That is your chronological age. However, your psychological age and your biological age can most definitely be changed because they relate to your mindset, and you can change that. There are also many ways to change your social or cultural age. Let's say you relocate - your environment or culture changes, as do your community and your social activities. Or, wherever you are, if you make a decision to change your behavior in spite of the surrounding mores (or because of them), you can change both your biological and psychological ages. You can actually control all of these aging categories except the number of years you have been on this earth.

Cultural change is something every family deals with when parents get older – medical issues arise and we worry about our parents living on their own. The aging process is winning the battle and something needs to be done. Unfortunately, all too often, the parents do not want to move and want to stay in their own home. My mother insisted she stay put, "You're not going to put me in one of those places!" Sadly, her stalwart position did not take into consideration the repercussions of her decision on anyone else's life. Nor did she anticipate the loneliness she would experience as the years went by.

And sometimes, while the transition to relocate to a community of similar folk is not an easy one, the reward can return tenfold. That's when we hear the stories of having found the "fountain of youth," where the parents meet new people and start becoming very sociable and active because of where they now live. Because communing with others is right up there with a healthy diet and exercise as a way to offset aging, they choose to thrive with new friends as opposed to being alone at home for hours and often days on end.

Have you ever visited a retirement or assisted living community? You can tell right away whether it is for "old" people or for people who live a life of vitality and just happen to be at an older age. The successful communities pride themselves on the diversity of activities they offer – both physical fun and mental challenges in which their residents can participate. Many of these folks are in their 80s and 90s and live very fulfilled lives with lots of friends and many things to do every day. The "culture" this life offers enhances their positive thinking, empowering them to believe they really can do more than they thought they could. The reality is they can - and they are! This "age attitude" keeps them young – both psychologically and biologically.

You will learn more about what can be done within these four aging categories. The goal is to keep both the mindset and the physical body in fantastic shape – at age 80, into the 90s and beyond. It really can be done!

SOME SCARY STATISTICS ABOUT OLDER ADULTS

This is just the tip of the iceberg when it comes to stats on the elderly:

Frailty
Signs of frailty are weaknesses due to muscle atrophy, unsteadiness, imbalance, tiredness, slowness, and, often, osteoporosis and/or shrinking.

Between 65 and 75, approximately 12% of the population is frail. Between 75 – 85, it jumps to 25% of the population. And over the age of 85, more than 35% of the population is frail.[2]

Chronic Disease

According to the Center for Disease Control, 60% of adults have at least one chronic disease and 40% have 2 or more chronic diseases. And 70% to 80% of those diseases are *preventable*. Along with those diseases come medications. Some medications cause side effects, which can lead to additional medications, which can then cause additional side effects, and on and on and on. This is how people can take 8 or 10 pills a day, sometimes more.

Heart Disease

Seventy percent of Americans ages 60-79 have some form of heart disease and 80% of those over 80 have it.[3] Most heart disease is due to diet and lifestyle and, therefore, controlled by the individual who gets it.

Prescription Drugs

Almost 90% of older adults take one prescription medication daily, 80% take at least two and 36% take five medications regularly.[4]

Alzheimer's and Dementia

In the United States, one in nine people over the age of 65 have some form of Alzheimer's and almost 2/3 of them are women. One in three seniors dies with Alzheimer's or another dementia.[5]

---

[2] *The Journals of Gerontology*, Volume 70, Issue 11, September 2015
[3] *ACSM Health and Fitness Journal*, January/February 2018
[4] merckmanuals.com, "Overview of Drug Therapy in Older Adults," September 2022
[5] alz.org (Alzheimer's Association), "Alzheimer's Disease Facts and Figures"

Sarcopenia

In the coming years, sarcopenia, or loss of muscle mass, will become a widespread public health problem that will affect 25% of the population under age 70 and more than 40% of those older than 70.[6] Believe it or not, we begin to lose muscle mass around the age of 30. Muscle mass decreases approximately 3-8% per decade after the age of 30 and this rate of decline is even higher after the age of 60.[7]

Isolation

"Studies have shown that social isolation and loneliness are worse for one's health than obesity – and prolonged isolation is just as bad for seniors as smoking 15 cigarettes a day…. Medicare spends approximately $134 more per month for every senior who is isolated compared to those who are not."[8]

WHAT HAPPENS WHEN WE AGE

Let's assume the aging process starts at around 24 and take a look at what actually happens with our bodies.

The body itself has finished growing and should not get any taller than it is. Our brains are fully developed. Our lungs and other organs are all now functioning at their adult capacity, assuming there is no illness. If we are healthy and remain healthy, we typically are not aware of the various impositions of aging.

As "middle age" approaches, we begin to notice some physical changes. Both women and men go through similar symptoms. It might be a little more difficult getting up and down off the floor or in and out of the car. Climbing a flight of stairs takes just a wee bit longer. We might start to

---

[6] nih.gov (National Institutes of Health), US National Library of Medicine/Geriatric Medicine, 2016
[7] nih.gov (National Institutes of Health), US National Library of Medicine, "Current Opinion Clinical Nutritional Metabolic Care," July 2004
[8] *AARP Foundation Newsletter*, Winter 2019

fade around 2:00 – 3:00pm and we want a little catnap to re-charge. (My mom faithfully took a nap every afternoon, starting at 62.)

Then, as time continues to march on, some obvious changes could show up in your posture, in your level of energy, as a random pain or achiness in the joints, as sporadic forgetfulness, as a newfound fear of falling, or as spontaneous weight gain in many different places. Overall, your body slowly begins to change and feel more foreign to you. And, as these aging years pass, your focus is more and more on these changes and the losses and fears they bring with them. So your mind jumps into the conversation, along with your body!

The following section outlines many of the body's systems, conditions and functions. It's a bit dry, but I feel it is important, not only to understand the physiology of these various body parts in the aging process, but also to recognize, appreciate, and perhaps be in awe of all that the body does for you without your even noticing!

Perimenopause and Andropause

Middle age is the onset for perimenopause in women. This interferes with the menstrual cycle and other hormonal functions. Our bodies literally feel different and change molecularly. There may be hot flashes, irregular menses and fatigue, but there is a multitude of other symptoms that can appear. Men go through a similar milestone known as andropause, although reports suggest they start after age 50. While men's symptoms are not always as obvious as women's, the testosterone levels do lower and they are susceptible to moodiness, fatigue, fat gain around the middle and the chest and an overall loss of muscle mass.

Cardiovascular Health

Our cardiovascular system pertains to our heart and blood system. Our blood vessels and arteries begin to narrow, making it harder for blood to move through them easily. Fatty deposits called plaque can collect along the artery walls and slow the blood flow from the heart. The result might be short-windedness as the heart has to work harder to pump. Remember, the heart's job is to pump the blood which contains the oxygen we need to survive. The shrunken vessels can lead to high blood pressure and a multitude of potential heart diseases.

Bone and Muscle Health

Our bones take a hit in their density which tends to make them weaker and more likely to fracture. Our muscle tissue shrinks, weakens, and becomes less flexible. As mentioned, we notice how stiff we are just getting up off the floor or out of the car. If you are a former athlete of any kind who did not stretch enough after actively engaging in your sport, your body might have a greater potential for tight muscles and connective tissue pulling in all different directions. This can be extremely painful and also increases the potential for irregular skeletal development – tightness in muscles causing the pulling of bones and joints in awkward and often painful directions.

Muscle tissue is known to atrophy as we age. We lose ½ pound of muscle mass per year beginning at the age of 30, which means we have lost 20 pounds of muscle by the time we reach 70. And, of course, the older we get, the less active we are. So, what comes first? According to the *IDEA Fitness Journal*, "Muscle atrophy in the elderly population is, in general, not a result of aging as much as it is a result of decreased movement over a number of years – meaning, people typically stop moving and *then* get weak, not the other way around."[9]

Digestion and Elimination

Our digestion and elimination system shows its age through an increase in acid indigestion or acid reflux, and an increase in the problems of constipation and irritable bowel syndrome. These have both become increasingly widespread as we know more about both disorders. They often affect people in their 30s and 40s, but with high stress these symptoms can appear earlier.

---

[9] *IDEA Fitness Journal,* May 2013

I actually was diagnosed with IBS in my mid-20s. I had a feeling at the time that the doctor really didn't know what else to call whatever it was that I had. There was no mention to change my diet, drink more water, exercise – nothing. No advice or suggestion for treatment except laxatives.

Bladder

Our bladder stands an increased risk of infection with aging. Urinary tract infections (UTIs) can be prevalent in both men and women. Loss of bladder control or incomplete urination could be evidence of holding it in all those years. This repeated practice has weakened and stretched the bladder out, creating possible pockets within the bladder that hold back some urine. So, when you go, you might not completely empty the bladder, and therefore need to go again within a short period of time. Potential side effects of menopause are incontinence and diseases such as diabetes, which can also lead to lack of control. As for men, causes of frequent or incomplete urination might be from an enlarged prostate, creating pressure on the bladder.

Brain Health

As far as your brain is concerned, your memory may deteriorate – more likely your short-term memory than your long-term. In less than 10 years for those over the age of 65, "at least 1 in 4 can expect memory lapses and fuzzy thinking, while 1 in 10 will develop dementia."[10] The potential for dementia or Alzheimer's is due to dying cells or cells potentially affected over time with plaque development. Other neurological disorders may begin to appear such as Parkinson's, ALS or Multiple System Atrophy (MSA), a horribly debilitating disease which does exactly what it says - slowly atrophies the body's major functioning systems, from the muscle system to the nervous system.

The older we get, the brain also gets lighter in weight and loses neurons, which lessens the brain's ability to send appropriate signals throughout

---

[10] *AARP Magazine*, July 2019

the body. This also impairs the rate at which you learn new things, even though the ability to learn is still intact.

Neuromuscular System

The neuromuscular system involves communication between the brain and the network of muscle tissue we each have. As we age, that communication gets foggy due to the weakening of the signaling between the neurons in the brain and the muscles' ability to read those signals. As a result, our ability to adequately sense the space around us can be more vision dependent and we can get confused, which can set us off balance. This can also lessen our coordination in doing tasks we are used to doing without a problem. We might notice our reaction time has slowed. Also, because of the weakening in communication within the muscle tissue, our muscles themselves become weaker.

The Senses

Our senses become affected with aging, starting with poorer vision as the lenses in the eyes age and possible cataracts or glaucoma develop. Macular degeneration, which slowly takes over the sight in the eye, has become more and more prevalent. As for our ears, it is possible that your hearing is slowly dissipating with the aging of your ear drum and the receptors in the ear which translate the sounds you hear. Hearing specific conversations in a room with a lot of people may become more difficult and continue to worsen.

Our taste buds also seem to wane as we age. They actually reduce in number and shrink in size. The foods that we once thought were delicious seem to have lost their appeal because they taste more bland. This often leads to a desire for sweet or salty foods, as we can taste sweet and salty more easily. This, of course, leads to more cookies and cakes or more chips and crackers and before we know it, we are ten pounds heavier!

Our sense of smell has more difficulty discerning different odors or identifying precisely what it is we smell. (My mom's nose at 97, however, was often much more sensitive than mine – good for things like smelling gas in the house!)

Skin

Then there's our skin! When we get older, there is a separation of the skin tissue from the underlying muscle tissue. The fascia and fatty tissue just below the skin tend to decrease in size and quantity. This makes our skin looser and more wrinkled. There are fewer and fewer natural oils being produced which makes the skin drier. Depending on the amount of time we have spent in the sun all those decades, our skin might give us away. Age spots, skin tags and wrinkles, OH MY!

Another potential impact to your aging skin depends on your lifestyle up to this point in relation to your sugar consumption. When you consume excess sugars, they can attach to your body's proteins. What results is a gooey effect on the tissue, especially in our skin. The results are more wrinkles and sagging skin. So, aside from the multitude of other health issues that excess sugar can bring upon your body, your facial expression and naked appearance can be affected as well.

Lungs

Typically, as we get older, the membranes between the alveoli and the capillaries in our lungs tend to thicken. Simultaneously, our breaths may become slightly more shallow, and the connecting tissues between our ribs become stiffer because they no longer need to stretch to accommodate larger breaths. Consequently, when it is time to make a demand on your lungs, you may get winded more quickly. And taking a really deep breath is much more difficult.

Sex Drive

Another possible transition worth mentioning is a lowered libido. For women, this often occurs with the onset of menopause, or even perimenopause. A lack of interest in sex coincides with the inability of the vagina to create enough lubricant even if aroused. This can make the act of intercourse uncomfortable and sometimes painful unless a lubricant is used. Needless to say, this can make it difficult when in a marriage or relationship. For men, that little blue pill seems to help out when the will is there but the body won't or can't cooperate. Another possible cause of a low sex drive could be medication that one or the other partner may be taking. Women may suffer from a fallen uterus or a dry or shrunken vagina. All of these can interfere with the desire for intimacy.

Body Shape

As we age, our body changes shape and movement seems impaired - a lot! Women's hips get broader and stomachs start to paunch out. Men tend to carry more weight around their waistlines. Our shoulders tend to round a little bit more and our posture is compromised. If you have been athletic in your youth and adulthood and have not stretched sufficiently, you may notice your legs feeling stiff, especially behind the knees. This means that your knees may be bent as you walk which causes a chain reaction in your hips and overall posture.

Eating and Diet

You can't eat as much as you used to and you seem to be putting on weight despite eating the same diet. Because your muscle mass is decreasing in size, your metabolism is slowing down which means you don't burn calories as efficiently as you used to. Consuming the same amount of food/calories and transitioning to a sedentary lifestyle will increase your weight.

Sleep

Perhaps you don't seem to be sleeping well. You might have to get up two or three times in the middle of the night to go to the bathroom. This disrupts the sleeping time needed to repair and replace your cell tissue, which is one of the many benefits of sleep. During the night, our body literally regenerates - billions of cells die and are replaced. The interruptions to sleep do not allow this function to occur as efficiently as it should, and we see the effects in every facet of our lives.

One other thing – most of us require more sleep as we age. In our 20s, 30s and even 40s we could get through the day even when we only got 5-6 hours of sleep the night before. But once we hit our 50s and 60s, we need 6-7 hours at the very least to get through the day. Of course, we should be getting at the very minimum 7 hours of sleep each day. Of late, as I approached my 70s, I have found that 8 hours is my new requirement to feel rested. Those in their 80s and beyond can often very easily sleep for 10 hours or more each night.

A Word About Telomeres

I am only bringing this up because you may have heard about them or read about them over the last few years. Telomeres are the end caps of each individual chromosome in which our DNA and our genes are stored. As we age, these end caps tend to get shorter and shorter. The shorter they get, the more we tend to become victims of aging and disease. Elizabeth Blackburn, President of the Salk Institute, is one of the foremost researchers of telomeres. She and her team discovered an enzyme, telomerase, that adds back DNA to the telomere ends as they wear down.[11] Which means that by strengthening the telomerase, you strengthen the DNA. The stronger the DNA, the less chance for disease and deterioration. This book is all about strengthening that telomerase!

Inflammation and the Immune Response

I could get into all the science here, but there are just a few key things to remember: Inflammation of the body's cells is caused by the body's immune response to protect it from invading microorganisms that cause disease. "Advantages of the innate immune response include the speed by which it can eliminate a potential disease-causing pathogen (within a few hours) and its ability to recognize and respond to a broad range of microbes."[12]

---

[11] *AARP Magazine,* January/February 2017
[12] *ACSM's Health & Fitness Journal,* January/February 2021

What scientists have learned is that inflammation is behind most diseases – from cancer to Alzheimer's, heart disease to asthma. In recent years, auto-immune disorders are growing in quantity and numbers of victims. Doctors are not really sure of the origin of many of these disorders, but high levels of inflammation to the pertinent tissue are very much present. As with all the other aging issues that can transpire, this, too, can be abated with some precautionary steps.

In short:

According to longevity expert Jonny Bowden, Ph.D., an L.A. Board Certified Nutritionist and author of <u>The Most Effective Ways to Live Longer</u>, "The aging process, including disease, loss of physical or mental function and the general breakdown of systems, is caused by one or more of four factors: oxidative damage (literally rusty cells), inflammation, glycation (excess sugar, metabolic syndrome) and stress. Collectively, they damage cells and DNA, wear down organs and systems, deeply damage the vascular pathways that deliver blood and oxygen to the entire body and even shrink brain size."[13] You have the power to take control of all four of these factors through diet, stress management and other suggestions you will find throughout this book.

There is not a body part, system or cell that is not affected by the passage of time. The important thing to remember is that regardless of this inevitable deterioration, we still do have some control. The pace of the decline and the quality of cell regeneration as well as muscle enhancement and tissue density are very much under our control. And the more control we choose to take, the slower the above aging issues will occur.

One other note: When all these body parts start to fall apart, our personalities can change. We can go from an upbeat, fun-loving person to a quiet, sad, bitchy and complaining person. As my dad got into his 80s and was dealing with a fair level of pain and disability, we all noticed he got very negative and tended to complain, completely unaware of his new mood. My mother told my brother and me, "if I ever get like your father

---

[13] *Natural Awakenings*, September 2015

is now, PLEASE let me know!" Both of us did let her know when her time came – she was about 93 and was very disabled and dependent at that point. Unfortunately, she disagreed and kept her sporadic unpleasantness for my and the caregiver's ears only. However, I noticed that if we could watch some funny TV, or keep our sense of humor up (we certainly shared some hysterical belly laughs throughout the years), her complaints were fewer. There are biological hormones that are released due to laughter which help with everything from mood to pain to frame of mind to disease. That's why a good laugh feels so good! Lesson: the older you get, the more you need to laugh!! It truly can be the best medicine!

THE NEWER SCIENCE OF HEALTH AND AGING

In the earlier days of medicine, it was decided that the body was a machine – when a part was broken, you fixed that part and the machine would be able to function again. The Western medicine system, in particular, is still very much set up that way. There are very few general practitioners as compared to specialists. The specialist focuses on that body part, learning every single thing there is to know about that body part. Certainly, how that body part interacts with the rest of the body is important; however, its relationship to the rest of the body is not the focus of the specialist. Often the medication prescribed could have an influence on other body parts, but that specialist's job is to fix the one part that brought the patient to him or her.

What is much more understood now in the functional medicine and alternative medicine worlds is the incredible interconnectedness that there is within our bodies, and the dramatic effect that emotions and stress have on our physical state. Physicians in this practice of medicine are mainly general practitioners. Yes, there are specialists. However, the whole body is considered when developing any diagnosis. And not just the physical body. Our mental health, lifestyle and how we handle our stress is very much a part of the conversation, the diagnosis and the treatment. Far more often than is recognized in Western medicine, an illness can be the manifestation of an emotional need that has not been met or psychological stress that has been going on for years.

Physical symptoms can arise, let's say in our shoulders. Perhaps polymyalgia rheumatica has developed, which I have certainly come across with many clients in their 70s and 80s. This is an intense muscular and joint inflammation causing pain that usually starts in both shoulders simultaneously, but can attack other joints and muscles as well. Typical treatment for this is steroids – sometimes for months and months, which debilitates the body horrifically, especially at an older age. Steroids do work, most of the time. But the toll they take on the body is extreme and can take months, even years, for the body to recuperate from the dosages.

If we looked at the disorder from a potentially emotional and psychological perspective, could it be that the person was feeling the weight of the world on their shoulders and they were feeling isolated and alone? And that perhaps this emotional drain had been going on for years, without any conscious recognition of it? What if we combined some psychotherapy and deep breathing exercises and meditation with the steroid prescription – at a milder dose – to help heal the pain and reduce the inflammation? That combination, along with a diet analysis to offset any potentially inflammatory foods, might just reduce the recuperation time. And the steroid dosage could be kept to a minimum with much less detriment to the physical body.

When treating the body along with the mind and spirit (often showing up through emotions) as a whole entity with intricate interconnected parts, it is much easier to see that everything works together in sickness and in health. According to Deepak Chopra, "the body and mind are not separate. They should be considered as one thing: the bodymind."[14]

EPIGENETICS

Through the most recent studies of quantum physics (in a rather obscure way) and epigenetics (in a more direct way), as well as through a plethora of scientific studies, it has been learned that we have far more control

---

[14] Dr. Deepak Chopra LinkedIn Post, "The Best Path to Lifelong Wellness," November 7, 2018

over the biological age of our bodies than we have ever known. There are so many attitudes we can embrace, behaviors we can adapt, diets we can consume and activities we can perform that allow us complete control over the progression of how our bodies age.

"The word 'epigenetic' literally means 'in addition to changes in genetic sequence.' The term has evolved to include any process that alters gene activity without changing the DNA sequence and leads to modifications that can be transmitted to daughter cells (although experiments show that some epigenetic changes can be reversed)."[15]

Genes are certainly important for determining the color of our eyes and hair, our height, body shape - our physiological traits that come from our families as well as what differentiates us from others in our physical appearance. When we are born, we are destined to turn out a certain way. If our parents had heart disease or cancer, we very often can "carry the gene" that could direct us toward that ailment. However, what we do with the physiology we were born with changes through our lifetime: We can become obese, we can develop poor posture, we can contract a serious illness, we can be prone to stress and anxiety - all things that are often driven by our environment and our behavior, regardless of our genes.

Former science, prior to the understanding of epigenetics, destined us to a cautionary life based on our genes and what they carried. We were doomed to be victims of whatever illnesses or biological traits our families passed down to us. In an effort to dodge breast cancer, women have had their breasts removed because they carry a certain gene that is known to exist in women who have suffered from breast cancer, and typically, their mothers had breast cancer. Children of parents who had Alzheimer's disease are plagued with the fear that they will get it, too. Same with Parkinson's disease or dementia, heart disease, diabetes, osteoporosis, COPD and many more. Just because your parents had it, does not mean that you will. Although there might be a lean in that direction from your genes,

---

[15] nih.gov (National Institutes of Health), US National Library of Medicine, "Environmental Health Perspectives," March 2006

according to epigenetics, it is your behavior that will determine if the disorder actually manifests in your body.

According to the American Association of the Advancement of Science, "Today, a wide variety of illnesses, behaviors, and other health indicators already have some level of evidence linking them with epigenetic mechanisms, including cancers of almost all types, cognitive dysfunction, and respiratory, cardiovascular, reproductive, autoimmune, and neurobehavioral illnesses. Known or suspected drivers behind epigenetic processes include many agents, including heavy metals, pesticides, diesel exhaust, tobacco smoke, polycyclic aromatic hydrocarbons, hormones, radioactivity, viruses, bacteria, and basic nutrients."[16]

Therefore, just because your parents died young of heart disease or cancer doesn't mean that you will. If they have dementia onset at 75 or severe arthritis starting at 65, it doesn't mean that you will. Whatever happened to your parents does not have to happen to you. Your behavior, your choices and your attitude are what will determine how you live the rest of your life, not your genes. So, the good news is that you do not have to be a victim of your family's disorders or diseases. The difficult news is that your future health is in your hands. It is mainly your behavior that determines the quality of your life in your later years.

For a thorough understanding of epigenetics and the latest theories and discoveries, research Dr. Bruce Lipton, a cellular biologist who has related the field of quantum physics with that of cellular biology, and in the process, created a link between science and spirit.

YOUR AGING IS NOT JUST ABOUT YOU AND YOUR HEALTH

As stated above in the "Scary Statistics," 6 out of every 10 adults have at least one chronic disease. And 4 out of every 10 have two or more chronic

---

[16] nih.gov (National Institutes of Health), US National Library of Medicine, "Science Advances," July 2016

diseases. (The word chronic means long-lasting.) Older adults with a chronic disease are taking, on average, four or more medications for that disease, more if there is more than one disease going on. And the cost of that condition is up to $3.8 trillion per year – much of which is paid for by Medicare and insurance, which means, it is paid for by you and me.

Perhaps you feel secure because you have been very diligent about your retirement savings and you will be very prepared financially for the years to come. There was a study done in 2016 which found that 1/3 of cancer survivors had gone into debt from their medical expenses and 3% had filed for bankruptcy. According to a Consumer Finance Protection Bureau study done in 2014, medical bills are the most common cause of unpaid bills sent to collection agencies. And about 20% of Americans have a medical claim on their credit report and/or currently have a medical bill overdue.[17] (At the time of this writing, legislation has been enacted where medical debt is to be taken off credit reports, but I chose to leave these statistics here so that you can understand how many people are in debt due to medical expenses.) By making the decision to take more control over your physicality, you could be helping to secure your financial future as well.

Or perhaps you feel that you will be able to work well into your 60s or even 70s. According to Ken Dychtwald, an expert on aging, "half of today's retirees retired earlier than they planned. The top reason people give for early retirement is unexpected health problems."[18] This could also disrupt your financial plans for your retirement.

If someone with a chronic disease is no longer able to take care of themselves, even if the situation is temporary, the imposition their condition causes on their loved ones creates a dramatic amount of stress, which in turn weakens the caregivers' health and enhances the possibility of their own future health being in jeopardy.

---

[17] *The Atlantic*, "Americans Are Going Bankrupt From Getting Sick," Olga Khazan, March 2019

[18] The Age Wave, Ken Dychtwald

NOW FOR THE GOOD NEWS: A LARGE MAJORITY OF CHRONIC DISEASES ARE PREVENTABLE!

That's right: 70-90% of chronic diseases are preventable based on the choices you make over the decades of your life – from childhood on.

If you focus on what I suggest in this book, chances are your aging will not look *anything* like the scenario I described above in the sections *Scary Statistics* and *What Happens When We Age*. Here is my truth to you: It is all about seizing control – making the decision that you will not deal with a body slowly going downhill, having to face one physical deterioration after another.

The potential your body has for longevity is amazing! Your body wants to stay vibrant and youthful for as long as it can. However, it is not in control over what happens to it. You are.

A study with 334,000 people found that introducing moderate activity can reduce your risk of premature death by 16% - 30% and, in another European study, it was determined that inactivity was responsible for twice as many deaths as obesity[19]

In the United States, according to the 2015 US Census, there were 47.8 million people over the age of 65. Projections are that by 2060 there will be 98.2 million in that category. Of this number, 20% (or 19.7 million) will be over the age of 85. "Some demographers have even speculated that the first person ever to live to be 150 is alive today."[20] The huge question that must be asked is, what will the quality of these people's lives be? What will the quality of *your* life be?

I lived with my mother for the last 13 years of her life - she died at 98. I can tell you with certainty, she had absolutely no idea she would ever live that long. Her physical condition was not good and she knew that. Had

---

[19] sciencedaily.com, "Lack of Exercise Responsible for Twice as Many Deaths as Obesity," January 14, 2015
[20] aarp.org, "Live to 100. Plan on It." May 25, 2017

she paid better attention to her physicality over the previous 40-50 years, her ability to move and be more active would have been far superior to the condition in which she lived. Hindsight is 20-20.

We *must* wake up to the fact that we all could be living a much longer life than we expect! The question for you to decide is, what do you want the quality of your life to be when you reach age 80, or 90, or even 100? You have control. By taking control of such things as exercise, diet, sleep and stress, your body can easily enter into a life of positive energetic health – no matter your age. Granted, there are no guarantees. And coming from one who understands at the deepest level that when it's your time, it's your time, I would still like to give it my best shot. And that is what I am doing with the multitude of choices I make every day.

I will say it again…
How you age is mostly up to you.
How you live and what physical activities you want to do are totally up to you.
How long you maintain your independence is mainly up to you.

My mother's generation was clueless - they didn't know they would live as long as they did. But we do. Ours is a better-informed generation when it comes to staying healthy. The choice is ours to make.

I am on a mission to help you choose well!

CHAPTER 1 RECAP

1) There are 4 kinds of aging: Chronological, Biological, Psychological and Cultural. We control all but our chronological age.
2) There are many scary things that can happen to our bodies as we age if we choose not to pay attention.
3) Our body is an intricate interconnected group of systems that work together to accommodate the demands we make and the functions we need to live.
4) The newer science of epigenetics has shown that there is a direct relationship between our genes and how they manifest their destinies in our body based on the choices we make in lifestyle and psychological stability.
5) How you choose to age affects not just your future but the future of those closest to you.
6) How you age is mostly up to you. How you live and what physical activities you want to do are totally up to you. How long you maintain your independence is mainly up to you.

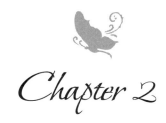

Chapter 2
EXERCISE IS A GIFT

"When it comes to health and well-being, regular exercise is about as close to a magic potion as you can get."

Thich Nhat Hanh

It starts as soon as we wake up. We sit up in bed, maybe stretch our arms out and take a deep breath. We put our feet on the floor and it begins - demands are made on our body.

We walk to the bathroom, we sit or stand at the toilet, we wash our hands and brush our teeth and our day begins. Do you realize at this point we have already used virtually every muscle in our bodies? Because this is our norm, we are completely unaware, but that is exactly what we have done.

I want you to do something right now – it will only take 10 minutes. Grab a paper and pen. Make a cup of tea or refresh your water. Now, think about your average active day. Make a list of all the things you do, from the simplest (like our start to the day) to the more extensive demands you make on your body: getting in and out of the car, driving – both short and longer distances – sitting at a desk, maybe being on your feet all day, going up and down stairs, going shopping, having lunch, running errands around town, picking up the kids, making dinner, cleaning the house or just picking up and organizing things, washing dishes, taking care of your children, your pets, your parents…. The list goes on and on. Write it all down. These are the activities we do every day without thinking about them. Please also make a note of how many hours you are awake in a day.

If you have an exercise regimen you can leave that off the list for now – we'll get into that later.

What does your list look like? Most likely, it is a long one!

Now, take a few minutes and slowly read the list to yourself.

How do you feel after reading it? Exhausted? You should - you do a lot! This little drill might seem excessive, but it is a real eye opener when you discover how much you expect your body to do.

The one common denominator in accomplishing all these things is how you are able to do all of it. Quite simply, you asked your body to perform and it performed as you asked it to. Unless you already have a physical issue, you don't give your body a second thought! You simply assume that it will respond to your commands to get you through your day. You demand – your body obeys.

So here's a simple question for you: Did you say thank you?

GIVING BACK

The purpose of creating the list is to provide an "aha!" moment in recognizing all that your body does for you. We are extremely demanding of our bodies and expect it to be ever-ready for us. It is only when we have an injury, an ache or an ailment that our awareness is piqued because our body is not able to respond as we wish.

We have to acknowledge our bodies in ways that show love and gratitude, as opposed to remaining blithely unaware of the expectations and demands we ask from it.

But first, you need to understand that the body knows.

That's right. The body knows when you are taking from it – getting you through your day, accomplishing all the things you need and want to do – and when you are giving back to it by giving it strength, rest, nourishment and yes, appreciation. Just imagine that the body holds an inner awareness that recognizes the difference between what it gets from you and what it gives to you. I can assure you, your body knows.

I can honestly say that in my twenty-plus years as a personal trainer helping people get stronger and more flexible, the clearest lesson I have learned has now become a favorite phrase to help my clients remember and understand this process of taking care of your body: When you give to your body, your body will respond to you in kind.

HOW CAN WE RECIPROCATE?

There are a couple of things that we can do. The very first one, and the easiest, is to just say thank you. Yes, sounds crazy, but it's that simple!

As I write this I am on my annual retreat. I checked in last evening, got to my room and started to unpack. I made eight trips up and down the flight of about 14 steps as I carried all the things I brought from my office and my personal belongings.

When I finished, I flopped on the bed, took a deep breath or two and said, "Thank you! Thank you, legs, for holding me up as I climbed and descended those stairs eight times in a row. (That was over 200 steps!) Thank you, back, for all that support. Thank you, arms, for carrying those loads. And thank you, heart, for remaining calm." I lay quietly and let my body relax and absorb the love.

We have a great connection, my body and I. It knows I am grateful for all it does; I never take it for granted. I recognize it and send it love multiple times each day.

EXERCISE IS A GIFT

The second and most obvious "gift" we can give our bodies is the gift of exercise.

Whatever exercise you choose helps determine the effectiveness this gift has on your body. The most important trait it must have is this: The *only* reason you are doing it is to benefit your body. I am not including any sports or other favorite activities in this recommendation for reasons that will become clear later. For this kind of exercise, my best recommendation is that you take one hour each day, six days a week, and give your body the gift of exercise.

I know, exercising six days a week seems daunting, never mind an hour each time! But, I promise, you can easily craft a routine that is not overwhelming, has a lot of variety and one that you will actually enjoy!

The seventh day is a day of rest – the body and the mind benefit from taking a break.

I am not telling you anything new when I suggest adding exercise to your lifestyle. We all know how important it is to exercise. What I *am* emphasizing is extremely important to understand: You must do a form of exercise that has no other intention or purpose but to give back to your body.

After we understand the best way to create a weekly routine, we will discuss the things you probably *think* of as exercise but are not actually included in the gift of exercise to your body.

My first suggestion for a type of exercise – and the most important form of exercise to do overall – is **strength training and stretching**. In Chapter 5, *The Unique BodSpir® Technique*, I detail the BodSpir® methodology – a meditative strength training technique I have created that allows the body to get stronger and more flexible at the same time. My clients love it and quickly see results. Because I cannot come to everyone, nor can everyone come to me, my website has an online membership program available for all, which is discussed later. You need to do strength training, and the stretching that goes with it, a minimum of twice a week. Or you can break it down into 4 half classes.

If a strengthening class is available near you, that's great! The social aspect of taking a class with other people can be a major motivator! Look for a class taught by a Certified Personal Trainer who has experience teaching your age group. Make sure you find a class at your correct ability level and please make sure that stretching is included in the class. Be careful with some of the strengthening programs that many gyms offer. They might look like fun but can be way over your ability when first starting out. Strength training does not have to be hard to be successful. It can be non-strenuous when taught the right way.

With two days devoted to strength training, you have four additional days to add exercise to your new routine. Two of these days should be an *aerobic* choice. That can include anything from a Zumba class to aerobic dancing or even a fast walk, pumping your arms to get your heart rate up. The goal is to get your heart rate above normal for at least 20 minutes. (We will go over the importance of our heart rate in Chapter 8, *The Forgotten Muscle*.) There are a lot of different choices you can make to reach this goal, but remember, there should be no other motive for exercising this way other than to give back to your body.

That leaves two days to fill with another form of exercise.

You might decide on Pilates, which is strengthening of the core. You might consider a barre class, which is a combination of ballet, isometrics, strengthening and stretching. Yoga is so very popular now, but you want to make sure that the level of the class is in line with your ability and strength. Another option is Tai Chi or Qi Gong which are both fabulous for meditation and improved balance. You might decide to take a long walk at a good pace, not to be confused with aerobic walking. In this case the duration of the walk is key, not the intensity. (As a side note here: I don't recommend carrying hand weights when walking. They create too much of a pull on the shoulders when you hang them by your sides for an extended period of time. Also, ankle weights are not meant to be used when walking. It can create severe back strain – this one I learned the hard way!) Maybe a bike ride is more appealing - again, you can choose between a slower ride or a harder one, depending on whether you want to use this as an aerobic day.

If you were to ask me which of these choices I recommend to fill your remaining two days, I highly recommend yoga one time a week. Yoga has many different forms and can be gentle or extreme. Talk to an instructor to help you find the routine that fits your body now – you can grow into other regimens. All yoga regimens offer peace of mind, breathwork and flexibility improvement. Yoga should not be hard. If it is, look for a beginner's restorative class or one that advertises beginning training. As you get stronger and more flexible from your strengthening and stretching regimen, yoga will get easier.

I take a gentle yoga class once a week. My body is strong and flexible because of the number of years dedicated to the BodSpir® program, so I can do any posture they introduce. The meditative component is powerful and a bonus!

When you get better at a new form of exercise such as yoga, you might decide to start doing it at home for 20 minutes or more a day. There is a multitude of websites and exercise programs to choose from online. I do recommend you take a local class in the same program if it is available. The class and personal attention can ensure you learn the right form and the right breathing patterns before trying them on your own. So many of us do not put our bodies in the correct positions and this can cause more harm than help. Be sure you know what you are doing – your body will appreciate it! Also, by attending week after week, you develop a relationship with the people and a commitment to showing up.

Here are a couple of possible schedules for you to follow:

Monday:	Strength Training	OR	Fast Walking (Aerobic)
Tuesday:	Tai Chi	OR	Strength Training
Wednesday:	Zumba Class (Aerobic)	OR	Yoga
Thursday:	Yoga	OR	Aerobics Class
Friday:	Strength Training	OR	Long walk
Saturday:	Faster Bike Ride (Aerobic)	OR	Strength Training

As you get stronger, you can change up the possibilities; just make sure that they are properly spaced. You should have a minimum of 48 hours (I prefer 72) between strength training sessions. Try to leave a couple of days between aerobic workouts as well.

The bottom line is that these suggestions, and the ones you find yourself, are choices you make for the sole reason to give back to your body, to get stronger, to become more flexible, to strengthen the heart and to show your body that you respect its needs.

EXERCISE VS. SPORTS AND ACTIVITIES OF DAILY LIVING

You might be scratching or shaking your head right now, thinking to yourself, "WAIT, isn't tennis exercise? Isn't basketball exercise? What about gardening or house cleaning? My body certainly can be sore afterwards, so isn't that exercise?"

My answer to that question is no, not in my world. Exercise is a general term encompassing many styles of movement and uses of the body. It is my intention and my passion to be more definitive.

Let's start with sports.

Sports are competitions in which we use our bodies to play certain games or reach certain levels of achievement, such as a medal, a trophy or at least a win. There are a lot of team sports: football, hockey, baseball, soccer, etc. There are also individual sports, such as golf and tennis. These sports almost always involve a competition and the goal is to win. In order to succeed, you use your body in whatever way you need to, doing the best you can to win the game. You are not focused on the body and what it is receiving – you are focused on doing your best and hopefully, winning. (Winning may not always be the goal; we may participate in some individual sports, such as golf and bowling, with more concern for socializing than for winning. The objective in those cases is to have a good time, not to give back to the body what it needs.)

In sports, you take from your body, you are not giving to it.

What about activities around the house?

When you do activities around the house, such as gardening or walking the dog, what is the goal of the activity? With gardening it's the garden and with walking the dog, it is to exercise the dog, not you. There are exceptions to dog walking. If you can walk your dog off-leash and you are both free to walk the pace you want, then you are exercising. But the important question remains – what is the ultimate purpose of the activity? Is it to give back to your body or is it to accomplish some other function and use your body to get it done?

> *Because of the mind/body connection,*
> *the body knows the ultimate purpose in everything you do.*

Sports and other physical activities are great, provided your body is physically able to do them. You should not be depending on them to get you stronger or more fit – that is backwards. Professional athletes know what goes into preparation – the concept is no different for you. When you give yourself the gift of exercising for the body, you will be much better prepared for your sport of choice or the activities you do at home.

RHYTHM AND ROUTINE

Another observation I have made over the years is that the body really likes rhythm and routine. It likes to wake up at the same time every day and go through the same activities as you begin your day. It likes to go to bed at the same time every night and eat lunch and dinner at the same time each day.

When you decide what your exercise program will be, assign certain days and times for each exercise day and stick to a schedule. Our lives are busy; I get that. However, as you realize the benefit this routine provides, you'll take it seriously and find the perfect day and time. Calendar it. Your yoga class might end and they are not offering another at the same time on the same day. What will you replace it with? Be consistent and develop the habit. Honestly, it took me a lot of trial and error before I came up with the best schedule for my body. We have found the routine and it works well for both of us.

Routine vs. Boredom

There is a fine line between routine and boredom.

Routine is when you are repeating the same activity of focus at the same time each day or within the week. Routine can keep you diligent and more inclined to continue specific activities on a daily basis. Routine helps us stick to a schedule and, ideally, get more accomplished.

Boredom occurs when you go through the same motions and do the same activity over and over to accomplish the same outcome, rather than changing it up. In my twice-weekly classes, each muscle group is exercised once a week. I have ten different exercises for the biceps, for example, so any given biceps exercise isn't repeated for ten weeks. That way, the body NEVER gets bored with how we are training our biceps, and virtually every tissue in our bicep muscle is being strengthened because of the different ways we are using the muscle to make the move.

If you don't change up the exercises you do with each muscle group, your muscles will get bored and reach a plateau of development. Just like you "tune out" when you are bored, so will a muscle. It will still do what you ask, but it will be more rote movement than charged movement. By stimulating the muscle with a variety of movements, you will encourage it to strengthen and develop the way you want it to.

Rhythm

One of the reasons why the BodSpir® technique is so effective is because it is strength training *in rhythm* with your breathing: the body's movement and breath are synchronized (more on that later). The ebb and flow of your movement and your breathing create a peaceful rhythm of body and spirit that your body loves. That synchronicity also helps make the exercise much less strenuous on the muscle tissue and yet still get stronger.

There are lots of ways to incorporate rhythm into your exercise. When walking, you can get a certain rhythm going with each step you take. You can keep a steady pace and count your steps in a rhythm of 1 to 4 or 1 to 8. There are walking apps with music that keep a specific beat going so that you fall into a pace that is steady and rhythmic. You could also add your breathing to be a certain number of paces on the inhale and a certain number of paces on the exhale.

The same goes for bike riding – you want to maintain the same cadence when you ride and can do that by shifting gears when going up or down hill.

Pilates and yoga, Zumba and aerobics offer their own choice of rhythm, unique to each exercise type. If you like swimming, breathing and stroking are natural partners as you glide along. Even canoeing or kayaking can have a rhythmic component.

The bottom line is to find a way, if you can, to get a little rhythm going when you are exercising. Not every form of exercise is conducive to it, but give it a try. It is sure to make the session more fun when your body hums along in synchrony with you.

Putting it All Together

When you go through your morning routine of getting up and getting ready to start your day, you are not moving your body identically to accomplish each thing. Your body is aware of the flow and can easily fall into line because you have established a routine and rhythm while you are on autopilot.

Find the "exercise" you enjoy and see how you can make it more rhythmic. I guarantee you that your body will give back to you even more! Keep in mind, movement in rhythm with your body helps you bond with your body. You are guiding the body in movement and yet allowing it to anticipate what will happen next. The rhythm sets you up for a closer connection and communication between your mind and your body, and if breathing is involved, your spirit, too!

A SMALL SAMPLING OF GROUPS THAT BENEFIT FROM THE GIFT OF EXERCISE

Everyone benefits from exercise, of course, but I want to point out that many studies have revealed strong evidence that exercise is beneficial for those with certain medical conditions:

TYPE 2 DIABETES: The position of the American Diabetes Association (ADA) is that, in people with type 2 diabetes, regular exercise improves blood glucose, helps promote weight loss, reduces cardiovascular risk factors (which are associated with type 2 diabetes) and improves well-being.[21]

CARDIOVASCULAR DISEASE: To improve overall cardiovascular health and function, the American Heart Association recommends a minimum of 150 minutes per week of moderate intensity exercise and 2 days per week of muscle strengthening.[22]

---

[21] *IDEA Fitness Journal,* July/August 2018
[22] *IDEA Fitness Journal,* May 2019

OSTEOPOROSIS: It is well documented and strongly recommended to do weight bearing exercise to help offset the bone loss that naturally occurs with aging. Although osteoporosis is more prevalent in women, men and women should get bone density tests as they age.

MENTAL HEALTH: "Associations between exercise and mental well-being have been documented repeatedly over the last two decades," according to the American Psychological Association. "More recently, there has been application of exercise interventions to clinical populations diagnosed with depression, anxiety, and eating disorders with evidence of substantial benefit."[23]

INSOMNIA: As reported in the AARP Bulletin, not sleeping well can have serious consequences for both our mental and physical health. A small but significant new study from Northwestern University School of Medicine found that a group reported a dramatic improvement in their sleep quality just by engaging in regular aerobic exercise several times a week.[24]

Overall, consider the fact that exercise gets your heart pumping, which gets your blood flowing, which spreads oxygen throughout your body, which is key to providing you with energy! What a wonderful daily treat you can bestow on your body - to give yourself a daily dose of oxygen to energize your organs, your muscles and all your moving parts!

IT'S NEVER TOO LATE

"The research shows that those ages 40 – 61 who begin exercising after years of physical inactivity can still extend their longevity. Even for those who have been couch potatoes for much of their lives, getting into a

---

[23] psychnet.apa.org (American Psychological Association), "Exercise Interventions for Mental Health," 2022

[24] aarp.org/health/conditions, "Sleep on This: Exercise for Better Rest," September 24, 2010

regular exercise routine after 50 can stave off premature death and add significantly to the quality of life."[25]

A FINAL WORD OF GRATITUDE

In the previous chapter, I outlined the different body parts and systems and what they do for you. I mentioned that I hoped you could get a sense of appreciation for all that your body does for you without you even noticing. The list provided was very short in relation to all that the body does. Just for fun, if you have a few extra minutes, go back and look at the list and the brief descriptions. Read the information with a sense of wonder: How does the body DO that? How does it automatically know what to do and when to do it? I don't know about you, but I find it remarkable and awesome – as in awe-inspiring. I am humbled and grateful – very, very grateful that my body knows just what to do and when to do it.

Think about the wonders of nature, such as the majesty of the mountains or the huge expanse of the oceans with the plethora of creatures that cooperatively live there, or how the rivers tunnel through the land to eventually find the ocean and pour into it, or the geese that somehow know how to fly in formation or a spider that knows how to create a web to catch its prey or the caterpillar that turns into a butterfly – the list is endless. Like the body, somehow these things happen without instruction or guidance – they just happen.

The concept of exercise as a gift to your body provides you with a new perspective on how you envision the partnership you have with your body. When you think about all you use your body for, doesn't it make sense to be in gratitude?

When someone gives us a gift, we want to return the gift in kind. It is now time for you to acknowledge the gifts your body gives to you, and consciously be kind to your physical self with the gift of exercise.

---

[25] *AARP Bulletin,* May 2019

CHAPTER 2 RECAP

1) We tend to make tremendous demands on our bodies, all day every day, without even realizing it.
2) We can give back to our bodies with gratitude and behavior choices.
3) There are several different ways to exercise which are gifts to our bodies and other forms of exercise which take away from and use our bodies.
4) The body loves rhythm and routine.
5) Everyone benefits from exercise, including heart patients, diabetics, people with weakening bones, people with mental health issues and many more.
6) The body is a miraculous group of systems and parts that work in brilliant harmony. It is of ultimate importance that we recognize all that it does with respect and gratitude.

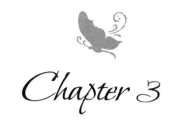

Chapter 3
EXCUSES, EXCUSES

"Change your thoughts, change your life!"

Dr. Wayne Dyer

Excuses, excuses. We all make them. Me too! In fact, let me assure you that I am the foremost authority on this topic. I have decades of experience in both making and abiding by excuses! Yup – I am a master at excuses, especially when it comes to diet and exercise.

As a matter of fact, I will make a bet that there is not one excuse that you have come up with that I have not! The advice and guidance you are about to receive is most certainly coming from an experienced professional excuse-maker – one who has mentally and physically found every excuse out there to avoid doing what is good for her. I wonder how many of these you have said or used before – and this is just a sampling of the most popular ones.

EXCUSES, EXCUSES FOR NOT EXERCISING

There's Never Enough Time!

The #1 reason people use as an excuse for not exercising is that they don't have enough time. Understood. And it certainly seems that it's an undeniable fact. Perhaps it's not really that we don't have the time. Most likely, it's that we don't have the commitment. Because if we had the commitment, we would find the time.

Let's break it down.

There are 24 hours in a day. If we follow the rule of good sleep, we get 8 hours a night. Sixteen hours remain. We work, we commute and we get ready in the morning. Fair to guess that is about 10 hours, including the workday? Now there are 6 hours remaining. We get home from work and dinner is a focus and we have to include time to get ready for bed. I am estimating we have 4 hours left now. For good measure we will remove another hour for miscellaneous things and we have 3 hours remaining in our very busy daily schedule.

How am I doing?

If you are like the majority of the population, You spend at least one, if not two or three of those hours in front of the TV, the computer or on your phone. Would it be okay to suggest that you limit your personal screen time to just one hour of your day? Even if you gave watching TV and being on the computer 2 hours of your day, you still have 1 hour available.

You are well aware that this time is negotiable based on your priorities. Many of us simply have bad habits – we know what we should or could be doing, but we simply do not do it. Do you ask yourself: How can my time be best spent?

Nowadays, your preferred television shows can probably be watched whenever you choose. The same rules can apply to your computer or social media time. Can you allow an hour for these activities?

Could you cut that viewing time down to ½ hour? How about 2 or 3 days a week instead of every day? If you could do that, maybe you could also add a half-hour of meditation to your routine, at least a few times a week to start. It's great for your stress and easy to do.

Many of my clients are retired or work part-time. When it comes to the "NO TIME" excuse, it's just not the true issue that needs to be addressed. The real problem is one of prioritizing.

Here is something you can do. Track where you spend your time and evaluate where you could find some spare time.

When I did this, I found that my evening hours, after dinner, were exactly as the research says – I was not doing anything I couldn't do another time – mostly TV shows or reading or catching up with friends or at my desk, working. I made the conscious decision that I would make an adjustment. By going to bed an hour earlier, around 9:30 pm, I could then start my day an hour earlier - at 5:30 instead of 6:30. I know it sounds early, but my daily workout now starts at 6:30 and ends around 7:15 – 7:30. PLEASE NOTE: This is what works *for me*!! You need to adjust your schedule to what works for you. Waking up at 6:30 or 7:00 could be exactly what works for your day. You need to find the time where it is most available to you. I do this five days a week and I am not rushed or trying to find time to fit exercise in. I also like to take a yoga class on Saturday mornings, so I did the same thing and arranged my Saturday morning schedule around the yoga class.

The added bonus to doing this first thing in the morning is that it is done! And you can feel accomplished for the rest of the day! That is a big help to my confidence and mental attitude – could be for you too!

If you already get up early in the morning so cannot add another hour there, consider taking that first hour when you get home from work or otherwise finish your workday. Do it before getting involved with anything else or you will get distracted, and what d'ya know… another day goes by. Put your workout clothes out, on your bed, waiting for you when you get home.

I have one stipulation.

Please, do not exercise right before bed. Your body needs a good two to three hours to relax from a workout. If you are exercising before bedtime, you will be doing more harm than good for your sleep cycle.

Here is the bottom line – if you really want to, you absolutely can restructure your day to find an hour for exercise. Yes – you need an hour. It is possible to break that down into 2 parts. For instance, rather than 2 one-hour sessions of strength training each week, do four 30-minute sessions and get those over with in the morning. Then, when you finish your workday, come home and take a brisk walk. That will be a great way to de-stress and greet the rest of the evening. Or perhaps you have time at your lunch break. If you get an hour, eat for 30 minutes, then walk for 30 minutes. Just make sure you stretch! Then, when you get home from work, you can focus on home and getting to bed earlier.

In the previous chapter, we learned that because we take so much from our body, we need to give back. The benefits far outweigh the "sacrifice" of your time. It's actually the *gift* of your time that will benefit your overall health!

Injury or Soreness

Another reason people don't exercise is because of an injury, or maybe when exercising they overdid it and are sore.

Injury is tough. Usually, with an injury, there is one part of your body that is injured. Would it be possible to still work other parts of your body? Any educated trainer will agree, there are always other body parts to be exercised, and it can be a wonderful coup for body parts that usually don't get too much attention.

Granted, you need to know which exercises to do - but that is just a learning curve, not an excuse to take a break from exercise. You can hire an experienced trainer, preferably one who works with people your same age and has faced a similar situation. Check with your physical therapist who will be able to tell you any muscle groups to avoid so you don't jeopardize the rehabilitation of your injured body part. Ask those questions, for your own health.

Do remember this, though, regarding injury: You will probably be referred to a physical therapist for exercises to help with your injury. Please know, physical therapists are NOT personal trainers and personal trainers are

NOT physical therapists. They each have their own expertise, education and knowledge in what to do in an injurious situation. Physical therapists are experts in the treatment of musculoskeletal injuries. Personal trainers are experts in improving strength, flexibility and overall fitness. Give permission for your physical therapist to speak with your trainer to clarify which muscles have been directly impacted by the injury and which muscles the trainer can continue to work on. I have spoken to therapists dozens of times about a specific client's situation. The cross communication is key in helping the client heal faster and not lose the strength and flexibility they had gained before the injury. Now, if your physical therapist just happens to also be a personal trainer, you are all set!

The most important thing to remember with any injury, the pain you feel is simply a way for the body to communicate that something is not right in a particular location in your body. Pain is a communication tool. In order to heal quickly, you need to listen to your body. Respect the limitations and let your body do its job of healing. Do the therapies that the physical therapist tells you to do, as often and as precisely as they teach you. Then, when you are strong and the injury is healed, *stop doing the physical therapy exercises*. They are not to be used as regular strengthening exercises. Get a personal trainer, tell them your recent history and get the exercises that will best benefit you in getting that body part stronger. Be respectful of the injured area, most likely for years to come. It is now a vulnerable spot that could re-injure. Go slowly and respectfully and don't overdo it or you could find yourself right back in physical therapy again, starting all over.

A side note here: I often suggest getting a personal trainer, not because I am promoting my field of expertise but because it is a very smart way to learn about strengthening and stretching exercises and how to do them correctly. Once you learn them, and you have a wide array of exercises to choose from and feel comfortable doing them on your own, by all means, let the trainer go. A key goal for any personal trainer is to teach their clients so well that they don't need a trainer anymore! So, when investing in yourself this way, know that the money expended is temporary. How much and how long you will be paying someone is solely dependent on your willingness to learn.

I Think I'm Coming Down with Something …

If you aren't feeling well and think you might have caught some bug, the flu, or even Covid, it's totally your call whether to exercise or not. I have studied diverse opinions on this and will share what I have taken from it all.

If you are coming down with a cold and it has not really hit your lungs yet, go ahead and do your workout. If your lungs are affected, I would not advise taxing them further with exertive aerobic activity. You might want to opt for strength training or stretching, as these would be easier on the lungs. The resistance you feel in your lungs is the way your lungs communicate with you that there is a build-up of fluid there. Forcing your lungs to do something more demanding will probably force them to resist more and scream louder at you in hopes that you will now listen.

If you think you might be coming down with Covid or the flu, or any other ailment that makes you not feel your energetic self, evaluate how you feel and decide if you want to put your body through a workout. Just make sure you pay close attention to your body's reaction to the exercise you are doing and if it just doesn't feel good, stop the workout. Focus and listen to your body. It knows best. And if you do have to skip a workout, so be it. (Look how far you have come in your enthusiasm for working out!) Now, let your body rest.

Common sense is the rule here. We are all different, so tune in to what your body is saying to you and let common sense be your guide.

AN IMPORTANT NOTE: The one thing everyone agrees on: Do not do any form of exercise if you have a fever over 100° - 101°F (38°C). This is because exercising could raise your body temperature and that can confuse the immune system – It will not be sure how to respond to your illness.

Aside from one week when I think I might have had Covid, I can honestly share that it has been so long since I had been sick, even with a cold, that none of this has been a problem for me. But, me being me, I am sure a long, long time ago if being sick were a good reason to not exercise, I used it!

I'm Too Tired!

For some this is just an excuse and for others it is a very REAL situation.

If your reason for being tired is lack of sleep or sleep issues in general, you are among a rapidly growing community – estimated at 70 million people per year in the United States by the Cleveland Clinic.

We will talk about it in depth later, but if you are not getting enough sleep, you need to slay that dragon first. Sleeping disorders such as sleep apnea may need to be addressed. But it may be possible to regulate your body clock so you can rest all night long.

Whatever the sleep-time hours bring, do your best to rest, if not sleep. Then, get your body up in the morning at your usual time to do a workout of sorts. Change up your routine a bit: include a walk in the fresh air, breathing deeply through your nose as you walk. Walk in rhythm. Also, reduce the poundage of the weights you use when on a strength training day. Include whatever stretching you can do, but try your best to maintain that hour each day to give back to your body. Your body gets used to it and if your sleep is not up to par, you want to do your best to maintain the rest of your schedule and routine to be as normal as possible.

Your sleep issues are quite likely to be caused by stress. Do your best to handle the stress and keep your routine going.

Scientific research has shown that even 10 minutes of brisk walking can help stimulate your body with more energy. So, if that sounds worth trying, do it and see if it works for you! You will be much more motivated to do the rest of your workout after the walk, or even just continue with your day.

I'm Too Stressed!

It doesn't take a rocket scientist to recognize that using your body in an exertive way, like exercise, is a sure way to help reduce stress. You are really using your body as a tool to eliminate the stress. It has been proven in study after study that exercise is also an excellent distraction to whatever may be troubling you, and, in some studies, even more effective than meditation, depending on the individual.

When you become a regular exerciser and are in a continuous weekly pattern of exercise, you notice that you just don't get as stressed as you used to. Things just don't upset you as much. If you suffer from anxiety or depression, with exercise you start producing dopamine and serotonin which are known to help alleviate these symptoms.

Let's say you had a hard day at work because a meeting you were going to run was canceled. Or your boss threw a new project on your desk and gave you barely any time to do it. Or, on the ride home from work, there was an accident and it made you 30 minutes late, which is now going to interfere with your workout time. Or the caregiver canceled and you need to find someone else to stay with your mom all day. All of these scenarios will cause stress.

But, as a regular exerciser, you recognize that there must be some way to view them where they will not cause nearly as much stress as they otherwise might. How can each situation be viewed from an "opportunity" standpoint? Your meeting was canceled, but you are now prepared for whenever it is rescheduled. The new project will give you an opportunity to learn new things and you will simply do the best you can with the time you do have to do it. As for the traffic jam, whenever I get in traffic or behind a very slow driver with no way to pass, I believe it is the Universe's way of telling me to slow down. So, I take a deep breath and do just that.

In other words, it could possibly just be a change in perspective that is needed to abate a stressful situation from ruining your entire day and then some. The more exercise becomes a part of your life, the easier it is for that new perspective to be activated.

Also, when you are a regular exerciser, you gain a sense of control over your body and your life. You gain confidence. You can handle things better. You move from an unsure mindset to an "I GOT THIS!" mentality! And because these are your new feelings, it is easier to stay in a good routine with exercise. The exercise supports the attitude which supports the exercise.

I Just Don't Feel Like It!

This excuse wins the prize every single time.

Believe me, I know.

I am in great shape because I am a personal trainer. It is my responsibility to demonstrate to my peers and to you, my reader, what being in great shape looks and feels like. This is a blessing in disguise for me, because the excuse of just not feeling like it can be huge to overcome!

So here are some tips that work to move past that excuse.

Give exercise 10 minutes of your time. That's right, just tell yourself to start your routine and only do 10 minutes. I can pretty much guarantee that once you start, you will continue to do the entire program. I have to use this sometimes too – yup, I can fall victim to this one! This works because it is not the exercise that is the issue, it is *starting* to exercise. So on those days that you just don't feel like it, do it anyway for "just" 10 minutes and I am pretty sure you will often decide to keep going.

Another motivation that works is to ask yourself, "what DO I feel like doing for exercise today?" Maybe weights aren't going to work today. Maybe you really want to do something different such as dancing or taking a bike ride or doing some yoga. Do whatever you can do so that one of your practices is accomplished and then you can get back on track with your regimen or schedule tomorrow.

The last thought is, if you don't feel like it, then don't do anything. Yes, you read that correctly. Do not do anything. *However* (you knew that was coming), what will you do with that hour whose sole purpose is to give back to your body?

Perhaps you want to prepare some dish you have been wanting to cook but haven't had the time. Or you might choose to meditate. Or you can read a book or article that will better educate you about your desire to be physically fit and in control of your own aging.

The point is, please do something with that hour that will contribute to your own healthy mindset and behavior. But you only get one "bye" per month.

The key to handling the "I just don't feel like it" day is to recognize that you are entitled to them. Believe me *(spoiler alert)*, I don't particularly like to exercise either! However, after all these years, if I take a day off, I guarantee you that I get right back on track the very next day. That sort of discipline came to me over time. I had to get the confidence and the trust in myself to get to the "knowing" that a day here and a day there will not interfere with my diligence. Again, starting is the hardest part.

It's Too Hard!

I can't tell you how many times people who have not worked with me ask me why strength training is so hard. My answer, of course, is that they haven't been training with the right personal trainer. (I am targeting strength training as this is where I have heard the "exercise is hard" excuse the most.)

There are many ways that strength training can be hard. The weights are too heavy, the proper form can be difficult to master, there is too little time for recuperation, the exercise itself hurts too much, and others.

Truth be told, strength training does not have to be hard. You can still get strong even when it is relatively easy. I am not saying that it's not exertive; it has to be in order to get results. However, if you start with the right technique with movements that aren't hard to do, you will find yourself energized and ready to move forward with your day in a very positive and self-satisfying way. And you will gradually become stronger.

It's So Boring!

I completely agree! Strength training is boring. That's why VARIETY is so crucial! The exercise plan I have created is specifically designed to avoid constant repetition of the same exercises so you don't get bored and neither does your body. The breaks in between each exercise with the appropriate stretch also help.

More importantly, the focus needs to be on the gift you are giving your body for all it does for you. So, when you are doing your iron pumping, recognize the dedication you have towards your future health. Be proud of yourself for doing what you are doing. This is your time for you. The only reason you are doing this is to help support your body so it can perform better for you. It's all about you, so allow that attention and embrace it. You deserve it!

I Don't Know Where to Begin!

This is a very realistic and popular excuse! It can last years, leaving you on the sidelines, never doing anything.

If this is you, it seems you are not able to get started on your own because of your inexperience and confusion due to all the information that is out there. That means it is time to hire a professional. By doing this, you gain a partner and an accountability coach who will guide you to success until you are ready to be on your own.

Hiring someone costs money. But being unhealthy and aging at the mercy of your inactivity is a huge price to pay later on. Is it worth the risk? If you know you *should* be doing something and have not started, this is your solution. Hire a personal trainer who is experienced in working with someone your age and with your physical prowess, or lack thereof. Beginning to exercise could be uncomfortable and awkward, but it should not be too hard. If the first workout is too hard, listen to your gut. If it continues and your trainer is not responding, simply pushing you to do the workouts, find another trainer. If you hurt beyond a 5 on a 0-10 pain scale for more than a day, your trainer does not know how to work with people who are in your particular situation. Find someone else. Working with a trainer can be a temporary thing until you have the diligence to continue on your own.

If you decide to join a gym, make sure you get some help and guidance on ALL the equipment. Do not set yourself up for injury. When I learned all the ins and outs of weight training, I was usually the only woman at the gym and was lucky to have the help of my fiancé, who had been working out for decades. When I decided to be a trainer, it was then that I did much more research to learn different exercises to keep the routines more interesting and motivating. A trainer can do that for you and with you. Your dependency on them will be up to you. Ideally, as soon as you learn how NOT to hurt yourself, you will be fine on your own.

Getting started takes determination and a belief in yourself. Do not give up. The rewards down the road are far greater than the temporary troubles that are present when starting. After just a few months, my clients have shared the following:

- "I could ski all day for the first time in years!"
- "I went horseback riding and, for the first time in 30 years, my legs didn't hurt!"
- "I went hiking with the family and could keep up with the kids!"
- "I went for a 20-mile bike ride and I have only been working out for 4 months. Granted, it was pretty flat, but still!"
- "I can climb to the third floor of my house without getting winded - over and over again!"
- "I fell down on my walk this morning and got right back up and kept walking."

I could go on and on with the countless changes that people undergo when they begin to exercise on a regular basis. So, please, ditch the excuses and accept the responsibility to take care of your physicality. Not only will your body feel better, but so will your spirit.

EXCUSES, EXCUSES FOR YOUR DIET

Having been a professional binge eater for decades and a sugar addict for most of my life, there were always ways to convince myself and give myself permission to eat food that was not healthy for me – to make choices that were the opposite of healthy. This is truly where I was an excuse master!

What changed in my life so that I can now adhere to a pretty strict, rarely-cheat diet started when I became a vegan. I am not promoting veganism as a lifestyle choice. It is not an easy choice to make and takes several hours of time each week for shopping and preparation. But I wouldn't trade it for any other way to eat. I am the healthiest I have ever been, and, as I mentioned, I don't remember the last time I was sick. I have been vegan for over 11 years now.

Adopting veganism as a lifestyle choice has allowed me the freedom to say "no" to so many bad foods. When I became vegan, I had already given up dairy for a couple of years. I had also just come off a 3-year relationship where I went out to dinner at least 2 nights a week at the best restaurants in the area and I had my fill of roast lamb, filet mignon and more. I knew it was time to make a change.

Most recently, I have become mostly gluten-free, and soy- or corn-free if it is not organic. (I found I have a reaction to glyphosate – the pesticide they use on these and many more plant foods.) I quit gluten, because I simply learned that there are too many horrific things about its physiological effects on our bodies and am now convinced that we all need to eliminate it from our diets. (I will give much more detail about food choices in Chapter 9, *You Are What You Eat*.)

So, with all that being said, there is no excuse available to me that would allow me to choose unhealthy food. You could say, I am excuse-less! However, as I mentioned, I am a master at food excuses, so let me just present you with some excuses that I have used in the past or that others are using with me right now.

Eating Healthy is Too Hard!

Yes, it is hard - but not <u>too</u> hard! It is all about choices - saying yes and saying no. Let's face it, we all know the basics of good food vs. bad food: veggies and fruit instead of processed foods, little or no sugar. But what about all those foods in the gray area? The ones that *seem* to be healthy, or the ones that say *"all natural"* on the box?

Here is the easiest, quickest way to *begin* to understand what a "healthy" food is. You have to learn how to read labels. There are 2 very simple rules to start with:

Rule #1. If you don't understand the words in the ingredients, it's probably not healthy.

Rule #2. If there are more than 4 grams of sugar in a serving (that equals about one teaspoon), you should buy something else.

Eating healthy is hard. It's hard because you often can't find much of a choice on the menu when you go out to eat. It's hard because people never know what to feed you if they invite you to dinner. It's hard because you often have to pack up and bring your own food if you are leaving the house for the day because there won't really be any place you can go to grab something quick to eat. (True to point, when I am driving a long distance and the only option is whatever fast food restaurant shows up near the highway exit ramp or in the gas station snack grab store, I have to say there is literally NOTHING that I will eat. Therefore, I travel with my own food!) Yes, eating healthy is hard and inconvenient. But I wouldn't trade my good health for a candy bar or bag of chips!

Eating Healthy Takes Too Much Time!

I completely agree!! One of my dreams is to hire a personal chef!

Here is the real issue. It is not that eating healthy takes too much time. It is the food preparation that takes time – and it does! You have to intentionally plan for preparing food to eat in a healthy way.

In general, I set aside every other Sunday to do my cooking. I will cook some of my vegetables for my morning green drinks and store them in one-cup glass containers then freeze them. I have one cup of vegetables in my drink each day - that's 2 veggie servings with a whole bunch of nutritious herbs, to which I add a half-cup of fruit and protein powder. I also prepare veggie burgers or vegan chili for freezing. I might make a rice or quinoa dish for the week or some other non-gluten grain dish. Once I started, I realized the possibilities are endless.

NOW the evening meal only takes 15 minutes – my prep work is all done! The time I spend that one-day prepping for the week saves me many hours if I were doing it for each meal.

Having enough time is really a question of priorities. If the food you eat is important enough to you, you will find the time.

My Family Doesn't Like Healthier Foods.

I have to be honest here. This one stumps me and stops me in my tracks. The 23 years I was a single mother, I did all the cooking. The kids ate what was served to them and they were pretty much stuck with what I was making!

I only bought organic milk, and we were on Food Stamps. There were no cookies or soda or ice cream in the house. The money I saved on those foods, I was able to use towards organic fruits and vegetables. We ate free-range chicken and local eggs. Lean hamburger and pasta with vegetables. If they wanted to have some juice, they had to go half and half with seltzer. Whatever junk food they ate, they got at their friends' houses. Birthdays were the exception, but otherwise it worked for us. (My kids might tell you differently, though!)

Healthy food is actually delicious, but it can be different in flavor and texture as well as in preparation. So, introduce one new food at a time so that your family is not overwhelmed. Perhaps each person in the house can prepare one of their own dishes each week so they are involved in the transition.

Take your time for the change to take place - do it over several months, or even a year. The slower the new foods are introduced the less threatening they will seem. Before too long, everyone will be used to having the healthier foods and the old foods are simply not part of your diet anymore. And, after several months of just the good stuff, go ahead and have a donut or some cookies. See how your body speaks to you after you eat it. Most likely, it will not be happy.

If, however, you are dealing with older children or a reluctant spouse, perhaps the key conversation should be educational and informative. Have a family meeting as to why you should all start to eat healthier. There is a plethora of nutritionists out there that would be more than happy to assist with this conversation, to say nothing of the tons of books and articles available.

I can share with you that the families who eat healthy from the time the children are younger do not really have any troubles in adjusting – I know of many families where the kids love broccoli, ask for cauliflower and really do not like the bad stuff. Remember that eating healthy and setting the example is a gift to your body. It is also a gift to your future health, which then becomes an extended gift to your children if your good health endures so they don't have to take care of you!

It's So Hard to Eat Out When You Are Eating Healthy!

Tell me about it!! You are not wrong! My friends always let me go last when ordering because I take such a long time and my order has a lot of details. But I want to let you know, not once have I been refused any request I have made. I carry my own olive oil with me to assure I am not getting anything with a vegetable oil blend. One time a chef came out of the kitchen to meet me and ask why I was so particular – I was very happy to share!

Okay – Here are some ideas to help make it easier. Order your main dish of fish or chicken or meat. When it comes to sides, ask for two vegetables instead of a potato and a vegetable (unless it is a sweet potato, of course). Eliminate the cream sauces and request no butter or oil on your vegetables. You can substitute lemon juice! With your salad - ask for the dressing on the side, then dip your fork in the dressing first, then stab the lettuce. You will use half the dressing without sacrificing any of the flavor it provides.

The key to being able to eat healthy when you are dining out is to be creative with the menu. You can mix and match anything on the menu. I have been doing it for years and rarely has a restaurant charged me more or given me a difficult time about my special requests.

I Want to Live Life Fully and Not Deprive Myself!

It is your God-given right to do so. Just keep in mind, you are determining the quality of your future and that future might not just involve you.

As humans, we share our lives with our family, friends and community. It is the quality of our lives that maintains those relationships. By ignoring potential health issues because today you want to "live life fully," you may be paving your way to dependency on those people you cherish the most. It's the daily behavior that builds a negative path over time. So be sensible and remember who else is involved when *you* "live life to its fullest!"

And guess what? An ice cream cone or treat every now and then is not what's going to sabotage your future self. But it may just give you a stomach ache!

Healthy Foods are Too Expensive!

This is an interesting excuse. If it is all about the money, what is your answer for the expenses you are going to have to pay at the other end of the life spectrum – medical bills, prescriptions, hospital stays and more? MANY more, if you end up with serious illnesses and physically debilitating limitations.

Do you know that healthier foods are more nutrient-dense? What does that mean for you? It means you won't need as much food to be satiated and satisfied. When you eat healthy, the need or urge to snack is much less, so you won't be spending money on those kinds of foods anymore. Think about it. No more sodas – buying seltzer instead saves a lot of money. No more cookies – no more junk food at all – saves both money and maybe your life! Take a serious look at how and what you have been spending your food dollars on and see what you can cut out and transfer to smart, healthy choices.

I am sure when you take a serious look at the foods you buy, you can create a healthier plan for stocking the pantry shelves and fridge. And if you eliminate the cookies, the soda, the chips and the crackers and use that money to buy everything organic, you could actually save money.

Let's talk organic.

When it comes to organic food versus conventional, buy organic as often as you can. It is more expensive, but the benefits are so important. And, I figure, if enough of us demand organic, there will be more available which, ideally, means the price will be more reasonable.

To save the most money, go to www.ewg.org (Environmental Working Group) and print out their "Dirty Dozen" and "Clean 15" lists. This list is a gold mine as it lets you know the foods you absolutely, positively should buy organically and the ones you don't need to worry about as much. The list is updated every year and the criteria for the food lists are determined by the level of pesticides/herbicides/insecticides needed to grow that particular food. Most recently, I copied their top 50 list of fruits and vegetables and organized it from most toxic to least toxic. I divided the list into two columns and keep it in my wallet, so when shopping and I want to check out some non-organic produce, I have it handy.

In my community, I am able to get organic produce, locally grown, every week, year-round! I know I am blessed and it is amazing. What I can't get from those places I can get from my local supermarkets. Many supermarket chains have their own brand of organic food now. Because they don't pay for advertising, it typically costs less than other organic foods, and they have pretty much everything you need. If you are not finding this in your area, write to your local market and let them know. Organic food is big business these days and I would hope they would be happy to help you.

If you are a meat eater, it is recommended that you eat free range, organic meat which is more expensive. But, if you cut back on the number of servings you eat in a week, you will break even by the end of the week.

One last thing about the high cost of organic: how much are you paying for a take-out meal for the family, or even you alone? Cut back one or two of those meals each month and you have easily saved the extra money you need for buying organic.

LET'S WRAP THIS UP!

I am sure there are a LOT more excuses you can come up with! Goodness knows I have! The bottom line is to recognize that while you might have your work cut out for you, it can be done. You need to decide the best approach for you, whether it's baby steps or one dramatic change. You are in charge.

Think of other challenges you have had in your life and how you had to adjust to accomplish them. I am sure you have lived through quite a few situations that were difficult, you thought you would never be able to get through them, or they were flat out devastating. But somehow, some way, you made it through. You got through those times and very possibly, have become stronger because of it. Whether you were a victim in those instances or the catalyst, now is the time for you to challenge yourself in supporting a future where there is no illness or debilitating aging.

Something intangible happens when we make the decision to take responsibility for our lives. We are no longer a victim, but accept that where we are is where we have brought ourselves. There is no blame, just a recognition of our role in our own life. The choices we have made have affected our bodies, our minds, our emotional well-being and our relationships. When we choose *not* to take responsibility, then someone else has the reins and we are at their mercy. It might be easy to blame others for our circumstance, but then that would mean that it is their responsibility to get us out of the situation we are in because we have given control over to them. But, if you are able to own who you are, warts and all, then you are much more easily able to change anything and everything about your situation.

What you will discover as you continue to eliminate your excuses and venture down the road of healthy living, is that your whole life seems to be blending better. Your mind and body are more in harmony, more in balance. Your body recognizes the efforts you are making and you are more relaxed because your mind is not feeling that sense of guilt for not doing what you "should" be doing ... because you are doing it! The angst and regret are gone. You're feelin' the love!

You are creating a future in which *you* are in charge of your physicality. No one else is making these decisions for you - they are all yours.

No more excuses, only gifts!

CHAPTER 3 RECAP

1) There are ways you can reschedule your day so that you have enough time to fit in exercise each day and each week.
2) It is of the utmost importance after an injury that you return to exercise with a systematic approach and not to just jump right back in.
3) There can be lots of reasons as to why you are not getting enough rest. It is important to establish a good sleep routine and schedule and stick with it. Your body will love you for it!
4) Stress takes over way too much of our lives. It is critical that we get a handle on how we manage our stress so that it doesn't manage us and take over our health.
5) Sometimes you just have to jump into something even though you don't want to do it. Chances are, once you get started, you will continue to the end. It's the getting started part that is the hardest.
6) As with choosing to exercise, making the right dietary choices are also just that: choices. You choose what you put into your mouth. And, although you may not think so, you probably already know the best choices to make!
7) It really is not more expensive to eat organically, especially when you eliminate sugary and salty snacks.
8) I have found that being a picky eater at a restaurant is well worth the conversation with the server and is usually cheerfully accommodated.
9) Paying attention to your diet is not easy and takes diligence and dedication.

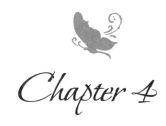

Chapter 4
MOTIVATION VS. INSPIRATION

*"Difference between motivation and
inspiration – Motivation is external and short
lived. Inspiration is internal and life long."*

Sri Sri Ravi Shankar

My first career was in the travel industry – the "incentive" travel industry to be precise. People who traveled on incentive programs had won the trip due to a motivation program that their company had offered. The host company would present a motivation "contest" to help their employees do better, sell more, or distribute more. The ultimate goal was to increase sales for the host company. The employees, salespeople or distributors were given rules, goals and guidelines to help them qualify to win the trip. These trips were typically to exciting locations and included amazing activities.

Their motivation came from their desire to win that trip - and often to be able to treat their spouse or significant other. Competition was among colleagues. Those who won were highly motivated to win and they took great pride in winning. The reward – the trip – was what helped them stay on track and eventually succeed.

The trip was their motivation.

MOTIVATION – THE DANGLING CARROT

Motivation is initiated by a desire for something or a longing for something. We identify something that we want and focus on it. Some may even pray about it. Whatever the goal or dream, it is always something that is seemingly beyond our reach. We are motivated to develop action steps to bring us closer to our goal. Every day we inch closer and closer to it even if it might take us weeks or months to achieve. Our motivation is the prize itself and our very strong desire for that prize.

The fitness industry suggests three determinants of behavior: capability, opportunity and motivation. Capability entails the actual physiological and psychological talent to perform a certain task. Opportunity has to do with the external factors that surround the individual, allowing them to perform the behavior. Motivation, as stated, is a desire for something or a longing for something. Theoretically, when all these components are intact, performance is successful.

When personal trainers develop a program for a client, we are continuously making suggestions in an effort to motivate our client(s) to exercise more, stick to a better diet, and establish a program that works for them. We help them set up goals and adjust them along the way. We also help them, if they need it, to identify their ultimate goal and why they are doing the behavior changes in the first place, if they do not already know. We help them fine tune their motivation.

You may have already heard of the S.M.A.R.T. approach to goal setting: **S**pecific **M**easurable **A**chievable **R**elevant **T**imebound. When you use these guidelines when designing your program to reach a certain goal, you are more likely to succeed. On top of that, the easier all these steps are, the more likely you will continue to succeed. According to behavioral science studies, this approach does work, especially if the goals are easy, achievable and done as baby steps toward a larger goal. Unfortunately, depending on the individual, once the goal is reached, it is not necessarily long lasting.

As personal trainers, we often help clients identify their unique motivators. These often include how to slow the aging process or to live longer, how to lose weight or get a better physique, how to enhance brain health or get out of depression, how to get stronger and be healthier, how to eliminate a disease or better manage a disease, how to lower blood pressure or decrease chances of heart disease. The potential list is endless.

There are many reasons people want to get better at exercise and diet - probably as many reasons as there are people! The real question is, *is their reason a big enough motivator to help them stick with a program long after they have succeeded?*

Sometimes people will want to start exercising because they have just been diagnosed with a disease, diabetes for example, and they know that exercise plays an important role in controlling diabetes. The real question is *not* whether it will help them or not. The real question is: What do they believe the exercise routine will do for them in this new health situation?

They may be terrified to now have to deal with this potentially fatal disease, but is that fear *strong enough* to motivate them to do anything about the diagnosis? Not necessarily....

"Every year about 735,000 Americans have a heart attack, and 210,000 of them happen in people who have already had a heart attack."[26] You could interpret that to mean that 29% of the people who have had a heart attack were not motivated enough to change their behavior, and as a result, had another heart attack. They were all facing death, but even the risk of death did not change their behavior. And 80% of heart attacks are preventable.

Even people on prescription medications for a chronic disease which could shorten their lives and/or diminish the quality of their lives are lax. "The treatment of chronic illnesses commonly includes the long-term use of pharmacotherapy. Although these medications are effective in combating

---

[26] *IDEA Fitness Journal,* Winter 2022

disease, their full benefits are often not realized because approximately 50% of patients do not take their medications as prescribed."[27]

For some, being diagnosed with a disease, and knowing that exercise and diet help, might be enough. They dive right in, hire a personal trainer and maybe a nutritionist and immediately get to work. They are hugely motivated to take control of their situation.

For others it will not be that easy. They might consult with a trainer for information, but not be ready to hire one. They might do more research and seek the bigger picture or anything else to put off exercising. The giant question for these people is, do they really see the exercise and diet change regimen as motivating enough to change their behavior. Unfortunately, too often the answer is no, they do not.

When the motivating force is just not motivating enough, there is not a goal in the world that, even if reached, will be adhered to. The fitness industry has completed hundreds of studies on how to motivate people and has created a multitude of theories on how to approach people, whatever their level of motivation. They have designed numerous goal-setting workshops and countless ways to get everyone – even those who have never exercised before - up and moving. But more often than not, no matter how successful the programs are, the failure rate far outweighs the success rate. These goals that are not reached, or that are reached and then lost – these failures are the biggest de-motivators of all.

This is by no means the fault of the industry. It is not the fault of the clients. It is not the fault of the trainers. It is the fault of human nature.

Being motivated can sometimes get us where we want to go, but once we arrive, can we stay there?

If we have spent decades being a little overweight or just a bit "out of shape," we very likely carry with us a little voice in our heads that might

---

[27] nih.org (National Institutes of Health), National Library of Medicine, "Medication Adherence: WHO Cares?" 2011

constantly tell us we are not good enough. And, because we believe we aren't good enough, the extra weight helps to justify that perspective. Because if we were good enough, we would be able to deal with this extra weight or this weak body. So, if we do get motivated and spend weeks or months or years working to achieve a goal, once we finally get there, we don't feel right with it. The voice still lingers.

In other words, the success is uncomfortable. We are not familiar with the feeling of pride in our accomplishment. As phenomenal as reaching the goal is, there is a letdown – and the "reward" seems inconsequential, because we feel we don't deserve it. So now what?

I can speak to this from personal experience. Aside from *always* thinking I was overweight, my battle with the number on the scale really became my biggest challenge after I birthed my first child. The night I went into labor with him, I weighed 210 pounds – after starting at 143 pounds. I had stopped weighing myself when I hit 198, at around month eight. After the delivery and getting settled at home, I was below 200 but certainly had my work cut out for me. And I was also dealing with a husband who wanted another child sooner rather than later.

To make a VERY long story short, I did lose 30+ pounds, got pregnant and delivered my second child weighing in at 195 pounds, just twenty months later.

Now I was motivated. There was no way I would consider the thought of having Baby #3 until I got my body back. And now I was the one who wanted another baby. It took me a little over eighteen months to lose 55 pounds. Again, I was highly motivated!

But when I stepped onto the scale and the needle settled at the number 138, I shockingly felt empty! This was five pounds less than my "normal" weight and I had not seen that number on the scale since my freshman year in college, more than 20 years before! Rather than being ecstatic and jumping up and down at my success of surpassing my goal, I was at a place that was completely unfamiliar to me! It was extremely uncomfortable not having to lose weight, when all I ever remembered, every day of my adult life, was that I needed to lose weight. I had *never* seen a number on the scale that was actually lower than I hoped for.

My entire life was spent fighting the scale, and now I didn't have that fight? Even though my motivation had kept me going until I successfully met my goal, there was something missing! NOW WHAT?

You see, motivation comes from wanting something outside of ourselves. Motivation has *objectivity* to it – the final goal or an object of desire. What I needed was *subjectivity*, something from within. I needed inspiration.

LIVING IN-SPIRIT (INSPIRED)

Life has taught me a valuable lesson. To live an inspired life takes more than just saying or thinking of something that inspires you. Living an inspired life takes awareness, acceptance, letting go, allowing, and trusting. It also helps that no matter where you are in life, having a clear idea of your reason for living supports everything you do for the rest of your life. On a daily basis, your inspirational life has no choice but to enhance your positivity and physiology throughout your body.

Coming from an inspired mindset pre-supposes that whatever you want, you believe you can have. Being "in-spirit" assumes a relationship and connection with God or the Universe or whatever your choice of higher power is. And if you do not believe in a higher power, you can be your own inspiration: Based on your life and the decisions you have made so far, you can be your own "Universe"!

When we become *inspired* with an idea or something we want, we tend to get obsessed (in a good way) with having it. We think about it a lot. We imagine it in our life and might even conjure up images of that thing, whatever it is, being present with us now – even though it has not appeared yet. Having dreams, and how we feel when we dwell on those dreams, can be our Inner Being trying to speak to us, bringing the idea or goal even closer to fruition. You might call this your soul or your trusted advisor – it isn't important what you name it - just know that your Inner Being is actively involved *because of how you feel.* When we feel good, there must be something very powerful about this particular idea, which is why we feel good. Our Inner Being is supporting us and agreeing with us through a positive emotion. When we feel bad or are scared or nervous, it could be that our Inner Being is trying to convey that whatever the thought is, it may not be the right one for us.

It's our emotions that help guide us to what we should and should not be doing. So, if a particular thought or idea or dream gets you excited and chatty, and lots of positive thoughts are conjured up by it, that's a good dream to have. You *feel* good about it. If, however, a dream makes you nervous or scared or wary, without an accompanying sense of excitement, that dream is not making you feel good. That's when you might want to take another look and re-evaluate that dream. If the fear is based on apprehension about the steps you need to take to get there, that's okay. That is part of the journey. But when fear of the *outcome* – the dream realized – is what you feel, that's when you want to take another look at the dream. Listen to the emotions that arise with the dream. If it doesn't make you feel good, that is your Inner Being telling you that the dream might be taking you in the wrong direction.

Most likely, this "want" is really strong and deeply heartfelt. You are emotional about it. Maybe your body tingles when you think about it. You feel a very strong bond with it, even though you are not living with it yet. The thought of not having it makes you sad. Again, your heart is touched by this incredible thing that will be entering your life. You feel excited and scared, but a good scared, all at the same time.

True inspiration is a gift given to you by the Universe with hopes that you will take the idea and move forward with it into action. You have a piqued awareness and, because it is something that truly captivates your senses, you can accept that this is your next step in life.

The best next step is to let go of the past and whatever you were focused on that was *not* in alignment with this new inspiration. And then you are on your way. Trust in the power of the emotion presented to you and simply allow it to be. You are committed and your destiny awaits you.

Pretty heavy duty, huh? Yes, being inspired is a *huge* deal.

Do you know that if we simply keep following our inspirations, we will evolve to the level of magnificence where we are meant to be?

So, what does all this have to do with living a healthier lifestyle?

Everything!

It is your inspiration that will keep you engaged in all the ins and outs involved in adhering to the program you are on. It does not matter what program – could be the food you are eating, could be the exercise regimen you choose, the water you are drinking or the meditation you are "om-ing"!

When you are truly inspired to change your life, the tasks that you need to tackle become easy and are now perceived as gifts that guide you to the life of your dreams. Your commitment to the goal is from your heart and is subjective. It's not from your head, it is not objective, as with motivation. Your inspiration aligns you with the life you want to live. And that makes ALL the difference in the world as you follow your path to what you have decided to be your success.

Do remember: None of this is easy. If it were, you would have succeeded by now!!

DISCOVERING YOUR INSPIRATION - YOUR 'AHA!'

Psychologists and "gurus" say that people will not change their behavior unless emotion is involved. As much as we may want to break a bad habit or change our lives for the better, unless we get a little spiritual or emotional about it as discussed above, chances are it will not happen. You may have discovered that being motivated worked for a time, but it just wasn't enough to keep you going. We can pray for the behavior to change, but if the yearning is simply not strong enough, most likely we will continue in the same old self-destructive or self-limiting habits.

Unless, of course, we have an "AHA!" moment.

For over 20 years I have studied with multiple thought-provoking leaders and had many "AHA!" moments. It is when those "AHAs" happen that our mind, body and spirit become one and we redirect our course of action to the next page or chapter in our journey. It is the "AHAs" that inspire us to change our behavior. It's the "AHAs" that keep us aligned with the new behavior.

So, how do you have an "AHA" moment when it comes to developing a healthier lifestyle? More importantly, can you create one?

You certainly can!

I am going to share an activity that is a part of my "F.I.T." Weekend Workshop. F.I.T. stands for Fitness Inspiration Transformation. We gather together and one of the first activities we do is set out on a journey to unveil and discover each person's individual "AHA" that will move them forward to a life of health and vitality.

This activity involves answering a series of questions regarding your future life. The object is not to just THINK about the future, but rather see yourself *in* the future. Place your mind, body and spirit in the future, feeling each decade as you move ahead in time.

Get a blank piece of paper. There will be columns and rows. In the first column you will write the questions I list later in this chapter; leave the column blank for now. At the top of the next column, write the decade you are currently in. If you are 56, for example, write "50s" at the top. The next column will be for your 60s and so on. Each row is for your answers to the questions I propose below, as they would be answered in each decade of your life.

You will need a chunk of time to do this activity, so schedule at least an hour on your calendar. You need to answer these questions from a heart-centered place. You want to give yourself the freedom of time and a peaceful frame of mind so that you can truly focus on the questions and the answers that come to you.

Here is an interesting twist of fate. Every time I hold a workshop and introduce this activity, almost all are hesitant and even defiant about taking the time to do it. They resist confronting these most basic questions about achieving happiness. It can be very intense and soul searching, and therefore, isn't it easier to just *not bother* to do it? I know that you have probably seen these questions before, but you have never, ever taken them to the level you need to. The process is tiring and it can be challenging to complete. However, every single person that has completed it has been elated with the results and very soon forgot the difficulty of the task at hand. They learned so much about themselves and their true dreams for their future. The exercise provided a roadmap through the decades and actually made them realize the future *can* last a lot longer, filled with an abundance of life – more than they thought possible!

I ask you to gift yourself the same opportunity. You are about to step into the future, decade by decade, starting with the decade you are in now and looking at it for as many years as you have left. For instance, if you are 56 now, start with the 50s decade and answer each question, envisioning your life from now until you are 60. Then proceed to the 60s column, 70s column, etc. The key mindset here is to become *you* in that decade. When you get to each decade, *be* that age and think about where you will be living, if your spouse or partner is still with you, and more. Become that 85-year-old so that you can feel the emotions you will need in order to make the decisions for your best life.

Extra tip: Please read all the questions through first so you won't repeat yourself.

I know you might get frustrated, and some of this might be hard to imagine, but I *know* if you do it sincerely and with your heartfelt desires, you, too, will love this exercise.

To begin, however, you first need to choose your Death Age!

What Is Your Death Age?

Most likely, this is not something you have ever been asked or even thought about! I am sure you felt that you have no control over when you die. I hope, by now, you realize you have more control than you previously thought.

That being the case, what age would you choose? What is your death age?

My death age is 104.

I was inspired by a sculptress from Ojai, California, Beatrice Woods, whom I came across when she was 104. She looked remarkable and vibrant (having now read her autobiography, she was!) and I told myself, "I want that!"

Many people ask me why I would like to live that long. Sometimes when discussing death age, people offer age 80 or 82 and say, "that's old enough. Why would I want to live longer than that?" My response is always, "Why not?" If you can be vibrant and healthy, why not?

Ah, but who's to say vibrancy and health are guaranteed?

As we all well know, there are no guarantees in life. However, I believe if you focus on taking care of your mind and your body, there should be no reason why your 80s and 90s can't be just as active and vibrant as your 60s and 70s.

Will you have slowed down? Absolutely!! But that is all part of becoming familiar with your body and learning how to communicate better with it. Listen to its language and be respectful of what it needs. It will be great fun to attain the age of 104 and see how healthy I can be at that age! Also, I am very curious where our world will be then…but I digress.

You want to answer each question within each decade of your life: depending on your current age, complete that decade as mentioned above, then go to the next and the next until you hit the decade of your death age.

The Questions: What are my Dreams and Desires?

What are my dreams and desires for my <u>career</u>?

What are my dreams and desires regarding my <u>family</u>?

What are my dreams and desires for my <u>home</u> and for my "<u>stuff</u>"?

What are my dreams and desires with my <u>friends</u>?

What are my dreams and desires for my <u>partner</u> or my <u>love life</u>?

What are my dreams and desires for <u>travel</u>?

What are my dreams and desires for my <u>spiritual growth</u>?

What are my dreams and desires for … *you <u>fill in the blank</u>!*

Remember, each question is to be answered differently for each decade.

Congratulations!! YOU FINISHED!

Please take a moment to breathe and to congratulate yourself on this accomplishment. We often forget that part. Enjoy the moment and feel the success! It was a big task!

You are now on your path to planning your future and we can move on to the next step. This, too, may take about an hour of time and it's where you will see the "AHAs" emerge. If you are not ready for this right now, make an appointment with yourself to come back to it. However, if you are curious and ready, go right ahead and roll right into this next exercise as the right energies are in place and your mindset is exactly where you want it to be!

This is where you can find your inspiration to take control of your physical future!

RECOGNIZING YOUR PHYSICAL FUTURE

Step Two of this exercise is to go back through *all* the questions and the answers you gave and ask yourself the following question:

**What will my physicality need to be in order
to live these dreams and desires?**

Let's say you decided you want to travel to India when you are in your 70s. What kind of travel arrangements are you envisioning? Will you be able to see all the sites you want to see? Will you be able to get on and off a sightseeing bus 15 times a day and climb whatever steps there are to whatever monument you want to see?

If you want to walk the Camino de Santiago (an ancient pilgrim route across France into Spain) when you are 65 to enlighten your spiritual path, will you be able to walk 500 miles in a 4-8 week time frame?

Think specific!! Be specific when looking at your answers. Quantify them even more to ensure you understand the physical demands that will be made on your body in order to accomplish whatever task is involved in your dreams. If you love gardening and want to keep gardening well into your 80s and 90s, how big will that garden be? Will it be raised or in the ground? Where in your yard?

When dreaming of visiting your grandchildren or great-grandchildren when in your 80s and 90s, will you be able to get down on the floor and play with them – and easily get back up? Will you be able to run around the yard with them, pick them up? If they live in another community, will you be able to travel to see them?

This is where the power of your dreams meets the power of your conviction to create and live your dreams. Will they just remain dreams, or will you recognize the changes you need to make in order to be physically ready to live them?

Are you ready to discover what truly inspires you and to take control of your physical future?

CHAPTER 4 RECAP

1) Motivation to change our behavior can often get us to our goal, but wanes after we get there.
2) Even when faced with life-altering diseases, a large percentage of people do not change their behavior to get better.
3) Motivation comes from your head; inspiration comes from your heart.
4) To be successful with behavior change, you need to become inspired.
5) Inspiration involves emotion and it is that emotion which helps support the change you want to realize.
6) If you could choose your death age, what would you choose?
7) By envisioning your dreams and desires for decades to come, you can often discover your "AHA," that which inspires you to do what you need to do to enhance your health and fitness levels for the years ahead.

Chapter 5

BODSPIR® MEDITATIVE STRENGTH TRAINING™ THE UNIQUE TECHNIQUE

"When the breath wanders the mind is unsteady, but when the breath is calmed, the mind too will be still."

Hatha Yoga Pradipika

When I decided to become a personal trainer, I knew I had to do it differently. I was 45 years old. I had been an entrepreneur and successfully launched two other businesses, each of those exceeding $1million in sales their first year. That was in the 1980s – ten years prior. There is nothing spectacular about veering off into another career path – people do it all the time. I wasn't nervous about starting a new business, because of my previous business success. I wasn't even nervous about shifting into a totally new field and doing something completely different. Those previously successful years as an entrepreneur taught me that I had to be unique. I had to figure out how to make strength training different without compromising its purpose.

I started exploring the different modalities of strength training to see where it could be unique – how it could be improved. How could I take the basics of pumping iron and make it a better experience for the body and the mind? How could I make strength training fun? Make it inspiring? How could I make it so people would look forward to their workouts? My research began in earnest ...

When I went to the gym, I was usually the only woman in the weight room. (It was 1997.) I watched the men with their variety of techniques of lifting and knew that what I saw would not work for me. I also noticed that not one of them ever stretched. That made no sense at all. After all the muscle contracting and the abuse their bodies had just been put through, they couldn't take ten minutes to realign their muscle tissue? I knew that was definitely not a healthy thing to do to their bodies. More research...

When I had a small collection of exercises spanning all the various muscle groups, I became diligent and concise with my workout. I paid close attention to my form and quickly recognized that when I wasn't in proper form, the exercise did not feel good. More research...

Many of us were taught how to breathe when lifting weights: Exhale during the exertive phase of the exercise (when you are lifting the weight) and inhale during the release of the weight. I was very precise about breathing correctly and noting how my body responded. More research...

Typically, we were also trained to stretch at the end of the entire workout. I started stretching immediately after finishing each set of exercises for that specific muscle group, building a lot of stretching into my workout. My body felt incredibly better than it did when waiting to stretch at the end of the workout. More research...

THE BREAKTHROUGH

My diligence paid off. As mentioned, an exercise has two movements – the exertive phase and the release phase. Remember, I was following my training and being very precise about the breathing while scrutinizing my reactions. I noticed that when exerting, I tended to blow the air out on my exhale and then, *suck it in quickly* on the release so that I would be ready for the next repetition. This would sometimes lead to light headedness and there was even a tendency to hyperventilate. Ever so slight, but it was there. It got me thinking...

WHAT IF...the breath were the priority?
WHAT IF...the exercise movement were controlled by the pace of the breath, instead of the pace of the breath being determined by the pace of the movement?
WHAT IF... the breath were in control?

THIS was my breakthrough moment. This was the "doing it differently" component that was unique! Instead of exhaling on the exertion, I was exerting on the exhale. Instead of inhaling on the release, I was releasing on the inhale. A subtle but crucial difference! The pace of my breath was determining the pace of the movement.

I knew that feeling stress, in general, was not a good thing for the body. So, why should strength training be stressful? What if it were more relaxing? When the muscles are called on from a relaxed state, they are less likely to be injured. When called on from a stressed and tight place, strain and injury are more possible. By "doing it differently," I had created an opportunity for the body to strength train from a more relaxed and less injurious position.

As I began to incorporate the breathing into my own workouts, I noticed a dramatic improvement in how I felt, not just during my workout, but afterwards. I did not feel as stressed and exhausted. Stretching after working each individual muscle group enhanced my overall flexibility. I knew that I had truly created an approach that can help people not just get stronger, but more flexible, too.

Now, what to call it? I will always remember the evening I was walking my dog, coming up the hill from the pond at the end of my street, and before I rounded the corner to home, it hit me! This technique is a combination of body and breath. Breathing - the process by which air is brought into the lungs - is also called inspiration. The process of breathing allows the body to be intrinsically linked to inspiration and living In-Spirit. The play on words was irresistible!! Body, Inspiration/In-Spirit ... BodSpir® was born!

I had created the BodSpir® Strength Training Technique focusing on strengthening and stretching, balancing and breathing, and hopefully, living "In-Spirit." "Meditative Strength Training™" became my tagline, a motto to bring the mission of BodSpir® into focus.

THE PACE OF THE BREATH DETERMINES THE PACE OF THE MOVEMENT

The breathing in this technique is what makes BodSpir® unique when compared to all other strength training programs. The pace of the breathing is the breakthrough I discovered in exercising for better aging. It IS possible to strengthen our muscles in a gentler, easier manner. In fact, many clients have said this workout doesn't really even feel like a workout!

Americans are reputedly very shallow breathers. Our lifestyle runs at a fast pace. Slowly but surely, we are beginning to understand the benefits of taking time to regenerate, to get grounded, and to appreciate that life is short and we need to take care of ourselves and take care of our bodies. However, that awareness doesn't necessarily mean we are actually doing something about it. To help with that transition, perhaps we could learn to take time to breathe!!

When I discovered the power of the breath in strength training, I realized that a second benefit from using this technique was slow, deep breathing – the same slow, deep breath we use in yoga and meditation. Now you can apply this beneficial modality of breathing to your strength training practice. When we take long, slow inhalations (preferably through the nose) and long, slow exhalations, our entire body calms down. These longer, slower breaths also slow down our movement.

In strength training, when doing a slower repetition, you will use lighter weights. With the rhythm of your BodSpir® breathing, you will find that heavier weights are now just too heavy to lift! You can still build and tone your muscle tissue, all with the added benefit of not compromising your joints when using lighter weights. The lighter weights are heavy enough when you go slowly. After all, it's all about the stress on the muscle, not the poundage of the weight! And more repetitions with lighter weights tend to enhance muscular endurance more than struggling and lifting those heavier weights. And it certainly helps to offset the potential for injury from the heavier weights.

When we focus on breathing, we become more connected to our bodies and give respect to the marvel of this human survival mechanism. When using the BodSpir® technique, you will take longer, slower, deeper breaths, helping to reduce stress. This will raise your level of oxygen intake which in turn stimulates digestion, improves fitness and even enhances mental performance. (See more details about the benefits of focused breathing in Chapter 6, *Breathing – It's Not Just For Oxygen Anymore.*)

I have to share what I believe is the best benefit you get when focusing on your breathing with the BodSpir® technique: It is being mindful of the experience. Your mind, body and spirit are working as one to help you get stronger and improve fitness. The technique actually becomes a form of meditation. You will move at your own pace. Deep breaths, slower pace, breathe in, breathe out, rise up, gently lower. Truly a unique technique!

Sometimes in class, clients will close their eyes and just get into it! And, because we all breathe at a different pace, everyone is doing the exercise at a different pace – marching to the beat of their own drummer, so to speak! Different people complete a different number of repetitions during individual exercises because they each have their own rate of breathing and, therefore, their own speed of movement.

EVEN LIGHTER WEIGHTS CAN MAKE YOU STRONG

In strength training, we are often taught that you need to bring the muscle to the point of fatigue to get stronger and build muscle tissue. This is simply not true. Strength training does not have to be difficult or strenuous. I promote BodSpir® as a "non-strenuous" technique that provides beneficial muscle strengthening. It can certainly be challenging, but it does not have to be hard and it does not have to hurt the next day to get results.

When you master the BodSpir® breathing technique, your movement with the weights is slower than it would be without a focus on the breathing. When going slower, you have to use lighter weights because it is just too difficult to use heavier weights. In Bodspir®, most women don't use weights over 10 pounds for any exercise in the program. These women have been doing BodSpir® for years, are all very strong and can pretty much do whatever activity they want. They can stuff their own luggage in the overhead bins when traveling. They easily lift their 35-pound grandchildren. They can do all those daily activities that require strength without worry because slower repetitions with lighter weights have made them strong.

One of my favorite stories is one my 90-year-old client shared, telling me that she emptied her jam-packed 30-gallon trash cans and hoisted them into the back of her car to go to the dump! Her feat was a combination of stubbornness, independence, BodSpir® strength training and some good ol' fashioned New England grit. She was so very proud of herself! And so was I!

By using lighter weights, we do not put the inevitable stress on the joints that happens when we use heavy weights. So, how do we know when a weight is too heavy? You can tell when the muscle tissue being recruited to lift it is just not strong enough, and you feel it – not in a good way. Or you are able to do the exercise, but you can only do a few repetitions. Or you find yourself using other body parts to help swing the weight up.

This is absolutely not necessary for your muscles to get stronger.

The system of using lighter weights and doing 15-20 repetitions is a less strenuous way to get strong. By going slower, the entire muscle has a better opportunity to be recruited. Going faster with a heavier weight tends to use momentum as an assist to lift the weight. Though 15-20 repetitions may seem like a lot, doing that many reps allows the muscle to slowly but surely get more and more stressed. You do feel it, but while the movement becomes progressively more difficult, the lighter weight allows you to continue and ideally finish the 15-20 repetitions per set.

A little side note about how many sets to do: In our BodSpir® class, we only do one set for each targeted muscle group. We do the 15+ repetitions then stop and stretch. There are many studies that have been done about whether two or more sets are better than one, and depending on the study, both answers apply: yes and no. For our purposes and the goals of your workout, one set has proven to be successful for BodSpir® practitioners for 20 years. So, it is safe to say, with this technique, one set is sufficient. (More on this in a minute.)

The key element is how much stress there is on the muscle tissue. You want to feel that the muscle has done something strenuous. You want to push your muscles and use them "past their normalcy," but that does not mean you have to push them to the point of fatigue. Going to the point of fatigue with strength training is hard and exhausting! And one of the reasons people stop working with weights is because they think it is too hard! Even *I* – a dedicated fitness fanatic – didn't want to work that hard, especially when it is completely unnecessary! Unless your goal is to get a great deal stronger than what you need to offset aging, lighter weights and more repetitions are the safest and most efficient means to get stronger for those of us over the age of forty-five.

ARTHRITIS, JOINTS, AND JOINT REPLACEMENT

Joints are junctions in our bodies where two separate parts come together for ease of movement and to enhance the function of each body part. They are mainly made of tendons (connecting bone to muscle) and ligaments (connecting bone to bone). There is also cartilage for cushioning between the bones. These allow our appendages to move in all different directions in concert with our bodies' demands.

Tendons and ligaments are connective tissue and can be strengthened over time with continuous strength training. Along with their respective muscles, they will slowly wear down from overuse unless they are being strengthened. When our muscles are not strong enough to accommodate the movement we are asking for, the joints will kick in to fulfill the movement request. Over time, this can be extremely detrimental to the functioning of the joint. The tendons and ligaments can get tears and lose their "toughness." Bigger problems can arise if the cartilage (cushioning) within the joint also wears down. This is, in effect, what arthritis is – the wearing down of the tissue within a joint, causing inflammation and swelling and consequent pain. When this has been going on for a long time, it can eventually create what is called a bone-on-bone effect. When a joint is at this stage, it can be very painful. When in the hips and knees, in many cases, a joint replacement is in order.

But the good news is, with proper diet, exercise and focus on strong muscles surrounding each of the joints, our joints have a fighting chance to withstand the chronic use and abuse we give them. They have the potential to remain sturdy, strong and flexible as we get older. This can be done through strengthening and stretching.

What I have witnessed over the last 20 years as a trainer is that when it comes to hips and knees, overweight people who do not strengthen their thighs tend to wear out their knees and/or ankles, and thinner people who do not strengthen their thighs tend to wear out their hips.

This is my theory and my observation. Building up muscle strength is key to offsetting arthritis and eventual joint replacement. The key to protecting our knees and hips is to maintain strong thighs (along with a proper weight.) Maintaining strong calves and shins is also beneficial, especially to the ankles.

If the muscle tissue in the thighs is strong enough to accommodate anything you request of them, then your body does not have to recruit the joint tissues to help you do what you are requesting. Always remember, your body is ALWAYS going to do whatever you ask it to, as best as it can. It doesn't think about what tissue it is using to perform the task, or if there is a potential for damage. The body just barrels through based on the commands you are giving it. Whatever tissue is being used will wear out if it is not strong enough.

Let's look at a real-life example. Say you climb three flights of stairs five times a day for over 40 years. Over time, because muscles naturally atrophy, your muscles weaken but your body is still going to do everything it can to get you up those stairs. The stair climbing is *not* a strength-training exercise, but rather an activity for which you use your muscles to accomplish a task. Let me clarify. When you climb stairs, the ultimate goal is not to strengthen your legs. It's to get to the top of the stairs, using your legs to do it. Climbing stairs is an *activity*. It is not an *exercise*. (Read more about this in Chapter 2, *Exercise is a Gift*.) Because the activity requires more muscle exertion than just walking, there is an increase in muscle tissue, but not enough to offset the natural atrophy that occurs with aging.

If the muscles in the legs aren't strong enough, the joints jump in to help accomplish the task of climbing up three flights of stairs. Repeating this activity for years and years, without giving the legs the strengthening they need to continue to accomplish the task safely, could ultimately wear out the joints. You eventually will feel it in the knees and/or the hips, and sometimes both.

One of the first aging challenges happens when the activities we are so used to doing, and take for granted, become harder to do. Our bodies start to feel it, but we continue, even though it gets harder and harder or the pain gets worse and worse. What happens next? In this example, most likely we have arthritis to deal with or, even worse, we are told we need joint replacement. In the early stages, maybe we just stop doing that activity. We take the elevator instead of the stairs and if those stairs are in our home, we plan our trips to reduce the number of times we have to climb those stairs. There are so many examples of how we scale down what we do. We do not play tennis, ride a bike or go hiking anymore. We can't play tag or even hide-n-seek with the grandkids. This is why most people can't imagine living healthily into their 80s. They assume they will start to break down!

To me, this is a shame, and for most of us, it is not necessary. The good news is we can change this! It is never too late to strengthen the muscles that are your lifeline to an active lifestyle. And for those just starting to feel these pains, the time is *now* to get into strength training to avoid a long and difficult future of less and less movement.

WHY IS STRENGTH TRAINING SO IMPORTANT?

Strength Training Increases Muscle Mass

Starting at age 30, we lose an average of 3-10 pounds of muscle mass every decade. This really adds up! By age 60, we have lost anywhere from 9 to 30 pounds of muscle. And, if you still weigh the same as you did when you were 30, you know what that muscle mass has turned into? The loss of muscle weight has been replaced by fat weight.

Strength Training Increases Bone Density

Osteoporosis is a devastating disease. Studies reveal that the onset of osteoporosis can occur in our 40s. It is a deterioration of bone mass, leaving holes and spaces within the bone tissue, making it more brittle and less solid, thus easier to break. This happens more frequently in women due to hormonal changes that increase the risk, but men suffer too. Osteoporosis tends to attack the spine and, in particular, the inside vertebrae in the thoracic region of the spine (the upper back section that is in line with the breasts, or a bra strap.) This subtly causes the inside of the spine to curl forward as the bone deterioration continues over time. We become bent-over little old ladies and men. It can also be extremely painful. My dad suffered from osteoporosis and we watched him shrink from a striking, tall 6'1" to 5'7" over a period of several years. I can still hear his cries of pain when he moved in certain ways and tried to do certain activities.

Strength Training Helps Stabilize Metabolism

As we age our metabolism gets weaker and slower. This is one reason why we tend to gain weight without really changing our diet. Because strength training affects our muscle tissue by making it stronger, our metabolism is enhanced and serves us better and more efficiently. We process our calorie burn much more easily and successfully. This, in turn, helps curb any weight gain and allows more control over our weight. Though the metabolic enhancements from strength training are not that high, muscle tissue burns three times the number of calories than fat, pound for pound. Which means, having weight in muscle tissue rather than fat tissue helps to more efficiently burn calories.

Strength Training Enhances Mood and Energy Levels

When doing strength training, the neurotransmitters in your brain tell the body to release endorphins. Endorphins make us feel good. You also increase blood flow throughout your body which circulates oxygen, resulting in more energy. So, you feel better emotionally and you have more energy.

Strength Training Builds Lean Muscle Mass

Yes, you will get stronger when you strength train. But, ladies, have no fear! Unless it is your goal, *you cannot bulk up!* The biggest concern of many female clients is that they will bulk up and look like a body builder, which is not their personal goal.

BodSpir® Meditative Strength Training™ is not the method one would use for "body building." Instead, the result is strength and flexibility achieved in a non-strenuous way. You will begin to notice a difference over just a few weeks. Over a bit more time, you will notice some contour to your arms. Certain tasks or sports get easier. But you could never come close to anything like the muscle mass increase of a body builder. If that is what you prefer, prepare to go to the gym 3 to 4 hours a day, every day of the week, and keep pumping heavier and heavier iron. (My guess is, if that were you, you would not be reading this book!!)

Strength Training Helps Keep Weight Stabilized

With a normal metabolism and a better diet, once you lose any unwanted weight, it is much easier to keep your weight stabilized when you strength train. Metabolism has a great deal to do with your weight and how you efficiently process your food. Because strength training is keeping your metabolism stabilized, it is also helping to keep your weight stabilized.

Strength Training Can Help Reduce High Blood Pressure

Studies have shown that strengthening the body helps to strengthen the heart (which is also a muscle), which helps it to function more efficiently, ultimately helping to stabilize blood pressure.

Strength Training Helps You Sleep Better

Studies have shown that another health benefit from strength training is that people tend to sleep more soundly and wake up more refreshed. But your workout should not be done before bedtime. Though more recent studies show that lower intensity exercise does not interfere with sleep as much as previously thought, I would still recommend 2-3 hours to rest after your workout before you retire for the night.

Strength Training Improves Balance

You have more stability and your balance is improved. This makes total sense. If your muscles are stronger and more flexible, they are better equipped to accommodate the movements you are requesting of your body. You lower your risk of falling.

Strength Training Improves the Quality of Connective Tissue

As noted above, when the muscles get stronger, there is less need to ask the ligaments and tendons to perform. You are not stressing them by overusing them, because the muscles can handle the strain of your movement requests. This relieves joint pain or inflammation.

Strength Training Gives You Confidence!

Think about it - when you are strong enough to do pretty much anything you want to do, doesn't that make you feel better?

It is a fact! There is nothing *bad* about strength training - it's *all* good!

MORE UNIQUE QUALITIES OF BODSPIR®

I hope you are now convinced that strength training is a critical piece for you to Thrive to 95! Here are a few other unique qualities of BodSpir® I have developed over the years.

There are many theories in strength training that seem to contradict one another. Some say you should work on several muscle groups at the same time and others directly refute that, saying you should focus on only one muscle group at a time. Whom to believe? Which method to choose?

Why BodSpir® Focuses on One Muscle Group at a Time

I know what works for the over-forty-five crowd. After 20 years working with people ranging in age from 45 to 96, I strongly stand with the theory that focusing on one muscle group at a time – first strengthening then stretching that group, then moving on to another muscle group – offers greater results, better physical range of motion and the ability to live an improved, healthy, physically active life.

When you focus on one muscle group at a time, your body has no room for confusion. It knows that it's time to work on the chosen group and no other. Let's say we choose the legs. Your mind, body and spirit are working in unison to strengthen those legs - all focus is on accommodating the exercise for the group of muscles related to the legs.

If you decided to drop some bicep curls into this focus, the brain would say, "Well, now, wait a minute. You wanted me to focus on the legs, now you are going to the arms. What's the priority here? I can do both at the same time - but not as efficiently as if I were focusing on just one thing." At least, that is what I think the brain would say!!

For that reason, the BodSpir® technique works one muscle group at a time. Then we stretch that muscle group. After that we can go to the next muscle group, pump iron, then stretch that muscle group. This way, all groups are created equal and get equal play – strengthening and stretching - within the workout.

BodSpir® Variety

The BodSpir® technique has more exercises than any other program I have encountered. I have selected 240 different exercises that have been divided into 20 classes or sessions. No exercise is repeated for *10 weeks*, assuming 2 classes per week. One of the common complaints about strength training is how boring it is. With such a variety of exercises, the boredom is alleviated and the curiosity is piqued by the thought of what comes next.

In addition, each muscle group is exercised in a different way each week - same muscle group, different exercise. This means that the muscle group is still being strengthened but the muscle tissue is contracting in a different way. This stimulates the muscle tissue to develop fully, and it doesn't get bored either!

It's Not Just About the Major Muscle Groups

In each class, we do 4 leg exercises, one for each quadrant, as well as 4 major muscle groups. We then focus on balance, abdominals and the often-forgotten parts, like ankles and feet, wrists, hands and forearms, and the neck.

Perfect Form is Important

You do need to perform the exercise in "perfect" form for two reasons: first, to get the most from the exercise, and second, so you don't injure yourself.

Long-term bad form can result in misdirected muscle tissue and joint pain. That is why a personal trainer is so important to make sure you are doing the exercises correctly. If you join the BodSpir® Membership Program you will see that I give intricate details of how to do each and every exercise to make sure you are in perfect form.

Good form when working with weights means you are diligent about letting the muscle do the work without relying on momentum. In other words, no weight-swinging when lifting. So many times, when I was working out at the gym, I saw people swinging their weights. They would do their bicep curl, drop their arm, swing it back then bring it up again.

The weight would be halfway up before the muscle had to kick in and do anything. The exerciser is using the momentum from the previous repetition to assist the next one, which is basically only doing half a bicep curl each time. They're cheating themselves out of the full benefit of the exercise!

With BodSpir®, we bend the elbow for the duration of our exhale, then, in a slow and controlled manner, we lower the weight for the duration of the inhale. That is our release. On the next exhale, we lift again, in perfect form, and lower for our release. Each part of the movement is controlled. At no time is anything other than the muscle tissue, in unison with the pace of the breath, controlling the speed of that weight's movement.

The 10-Week Conclusive BodSpir® Experience

Within those ten weeks of completing 240 exercises with no repeated exercises, we don't just work on "major" muscles groups. We know as aging adults that there are a lot more body parts to focus on as we get older. So, we work and stretch the neck, hands and wrists, even the ankles and toes. Everything gets strengthened and stretched. Your body loves it and is much stronger and more flexible because of it.

After those first 10 weeks, then you start over again with Class One, realizing the weights you used for the classes when you started now need to be increased, as you have gotten that much stronger!

There is NO Competition – Except with Yourself!

BodSpir® members and clients leave their competitive hats at the door. With BodSpir®, it is *NOT* about how heavy a weight you are lifting. It is *NOT* about how many reps you complete in a cycle.

It *IS* about what your body feels when it lifts a weight. The number on the weight is simply the identification of what weight to use when performing that particular exercise or working that particular muscle group. You could be lifting a 3-pound weight or 7-pound weight. The only thing that matters is HOW it stresses your muscle.

THE UNIQUE BODSPIR® TECHNIQUE

As you can see, BodSpir®, or Meditative Strength Training™, is truly a unique strength-training technique.

Over the years I have taught thousands and thousands of classes and worked with many individuals, all aged 45 to 90+. The biggest bonus I realized in creating this methodology is that strength training can also be a meditative practice.

One definition of *inspiration* is the process by which air is brought into the lungs. When you move your body in rhythm with your breathing, a synergy of body and breath (or inspiration) is created. To be able to give the gift of stronger muscles and more flexible tissue to your body, you are well on your way to an enhanced lifestyle for decades to come.

CHAPTER 5 RECAP

1) BodSpir® Meditative Strength Training™ was created as a variation on a theme of regular strength training, covering the major muscle groups and the smaller, often forgotten muscles, too.
2) The four cornerstones of BodSpir® are strengthening and stretching, balancing and breathing.
3) In traditional strength training, you exhale during the exertion phase and inhale on the release. With BodSpir®, you time your exertion to your exhale and time your release to your inhale.
4) The pace of the breath determines the pace of the movement which allows for slower, deeper breathing. When you breathe slower, you use lighter weights. With lighter weights, you put less stress on the joints.
5) There are many benefits to strength training, such as increasing bone mass, enhancing your mood, better sleep, controlling weight gain or assisting with weight loss, balance and more.
6) BodSpir® offers the unique option of meditation in conjunction with your strength training workout.

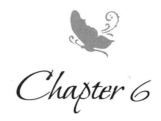

Chapter 6

BREATHING: IT'S NOT JUST FOR OXYGEN ANYMORE

*When one gives undivided attention to the
(vital) breath and brings it to the utmost degree
of pliancy, he can become as a tender babe.*

LaoTzu, the Tao Te Ching

Breathe in…breathe out…breathe in…breathe out…. The most critical subconscious behavior we engage in each and every minute. Actually 10 to 20+ times per minute, and up to 60 times per minute in a stressful situation.

The reason we breathe is to intake air and extract oxygen from it. Oxygen is the most vital commodity to our survival. Without it we would only last a few minutes – maybe three – or suffer severe brain damage if deprived too long and live through it.

There are exceptions to that statement. For instance, freediving is a sport that has been around for centuries. Way back when, it was done for food or for gathering sponges or pearls or other treasures for trading. Nowadays it is more of a competitive thing, with numerous men and women striving to set the next world record to depths as deep as 700 feet, holding their breath for as long as 10 minutes. Needless to say, these are well practiced individuals who enjoy the challenge of the dive.

But for most of us, oxygen deprivation for more than 3 minutes could cause some serious harm. Upon our inhale, the oxygen enters our lungs through our trachea, goes into our bronchi and into our bronchioles to our alveoli, where the tissue is so thin it combines with our capillaries and the exchange of oxygen for carbon dioxide takes place. The oxygen fuels our body and the carbon dioxide is the waste product from that fueling. None of this is new information. What is new is the increased awareness in mainstream America in the last 50 years (though much of the rest of the world is already aware) that there are many different ways to control your breathing which, in turn, can help control your stress and your health.

There are now hundreds of books in circulation about breathing from hundreds of different authors who discuss hundreds of different ways to breathe, each with their own specific techniques and benefits. I have listed a handful of authors at the end of this chapter if you want to dive deeper, no pun intended. For the purpose of helping to control your stress and your health, I will present just a few practices to get you started and/or curious. I have used all of these and presently usually combine a couple of them during my meditation and throughout my day.

NASAL BREATHING

Nasal breathing, needless to say, is breathing through the nose. The inhale is the most critical part of nasal breathing, which is logical. After all, the nose is equipped with nasal hairs which act as filters to help protect the body from germs, toxins, bacteria, smog and pathogens in general. Ironically, even though these nose hairs are obviously there for a purpose, no one bothers to teach us that we should breathe through our nose because it is logically healthier for us.

The real secret behind nasal breathing, though, is that the passageway for the air is so small compared to the mouth, it takes us longer to inhale and exhale. Taking longer to breathe automatically slows us down and helps to de-stress the body and the mind.

Nasal tissue is similar to muscle tissue. If you use it regularly it will stay toned. If you don't use it, it can atrophy and lose flexibility and tone. When this happens, congestion can ensue and a whole list of issues can be triggered. The most obvious conditions that can arise are snoring and sleep apnea – the condition whereby your breathing stops and starts while you are sleeping.

There have been a few studies done where people who close their mouths while sleeping (typically by taping their mouth shut) have fewer instances of sleep apnea and can sleep through the night, potentially eliminating the issues that sleep apnea creates, such as fatigue, grogginess, foggy brain, dry mouth and bad breath. There has also been a link from sleep apnea to heart conditions, atrial fibrillation, high blood pressure and risk of stroke.

"Proponents of mouth taping claim it may help reduce the negative effects thought to be associated with mouth breathing, including:

- Attention deficit hyperactivity disorder (ADHD) symptoms
- Sleep-disordered breathing
- Dry mouth
- Cavities
- Gum disease
- Bad breath
- Slowed growth in children
- Decreased cognitive ability" [28]

I hope that the Western medical community chooses to do more research with mouth taping. Think of how much money people could save if, in fact, it were as effective as the CPAP machine, which is commonly prescribed for those who suffer from sleep apnea. And think of the better nights' sleep couples would get when one suffers from this condition and has to use the machine, which can be noisy and uncomfortable. In the

---

[28] sleepfoundation.org, "Mouth Taping for Sleep"

meantime, I would discuss any changes to your sleep habits with your doctor before venturing forth on your own.

Another benefit of nasal breathing is that "nasal breathing alone can boost nitric oxide sixfold, which is one of the reasons we can absorb about 18 percent more oxygen than by just breathing through the mouth."[29] This is because nitric oxide affects the body by opening and constricting the blood vessels more easily, which helps our cardiovascular system, blood pressure, relaxation response, inflammation, athletic performance and a plethora of other good things. All from simply breathing through your nose rather than your mouth.

Here's something you can easily try yourself: Next time you are feeling a bit nervous or anxious, try to slow yourself down by consciously breathing, inhaling and exhaling, through your nose. If you are in traffic and feeling frustrated, do some nasal breathing. If someone has upset you or you get angry at a situation, do some nasal breathing. If you are waiting for an important phone call and your anxiety rises while you wait, do some nasal breathing. By doing this simple breath source change, you might find that your anxiety begins to wane, anger begins to subside, and angst in a situation eases. Try it!

If I haven't convinced you yet to pay attention to breathing more frequently through your nose, I suggest you look it up by entering "benefits of nose breathing vs. mouth breathing" into your search engine. You will find that the benefits of nose breathing far outweigh the minimal benefits of mouth breathing.

I, for one, have recently begun mouth taping while I sleep at night. I have been known to snore on occasion and, rarely, have experienced the gasp of sleep apnea. I can tell you this, I had no trouble adapting to the tape on my mouth, except when I would want a sip of water in the middle of the night. I also have found that if I do have to get up in the middle of the night, I am falling right back to sleep, which rarely used to happen. I look forward to noticing other benefits as time goes on. One thing is for sure: I am now non-stop nasal breathing for 7-8 hours a day, and that's a good thing!

---

[29] *Breath – The New Science of a Lost Art*, James Nestor

DIAPHRAGMATIC OR DEEP BREATHING

The diaphragm is the dome-shaped muscle that lies below our lungs. Whether we notice or not, the diaphragm bellows down towards our lower torso upon inhaling and rises and arcs upwards towards our lungs when we exhale. As we age, as with all muscles unless exercised, the diaphragm atrophies. It continues going up and down, but not with as much verve as in our younger years. So, as time goes on, our breath becomes shallower, and consequently our oxygen intake decreases.

Enter diaphragmatic breathing. Diaphragmatic breathing is a conscious effort to push the diaphragm down on your inhale, allowing it to arc deeply into the lower torso. This expands the capacity of the lungs, allowing us to take in more oxygen. On your exhale, you gently arch the diaphragm higher towards the lungs, forcing more air out of the lungs. By thinking about and performing your breathing in this manner, you are giving your diaphragm a good workout, allowing it to extend and contract to the maximum of its ability, which also enhances the oxygen/carbon dioxide exchange in your lungs.

By consciously using our diaphragm while breathing, we are helping the heart do its job of circulating the oxygen throughout the body in exchange for carbon dioxide which the lungs release back into the atmosphere. Keep in mind that the heart, too, is a muscle, and if it has to do all the work, it can fatigue more easily. If the majority of your breathing is typically with shallow breaths, you are only using a very small percentage of your diaphragm's purpose and ability. It is there to help your heart with breathing and it makes sense for us to pay much more attention to it. It could help stave off high blood pressure and/or circulation problems.

It might seem awkward trying to control this movement of your diaphragm, but if you concentrate on slowly pushing the diaphragm down and raising it up, it will make a real difference.

IMPORTANT NOTE: Each time you push the diaphragm down, your stomach will naturally distend, but your conscious effort should be to push the diaphragm down towards the pelvic floor, *not* to stick out your stomach. (Just breathing and sticking the stomach out can be done with shallow breathing, so you may not be getting the full effect of an expanded diaphragm.)

I have found diaphragmatic breathing to be immensely helpful with my focus while meditating. I take slow inhales through my nose, allowing my diaphragm to expand to its maximum, and then I slowly release the breath, still through my nose, and force the diaphragm as high into the lungs as is comfortable. By doing this, I take fewer than 2 breaths per minute. A wonderfully relaxing way to meditate and do even more than just relieve stress.

SLOW BREATHING

There is nothing surprising about what slow breathing is – it is making a conscious effort to breathe slowly. It is not necessarily deep breathing or diaphragmatic breathing. It is simply focusing on each breath, taking it in slowly through the nose, and releasing it slowly either through the nose or the mouth.

Slow breathing comes in handy when you are feeling a bit stressed about something and need to calm down. Or, you are faced with a decision to make and you are not quite sure what to do. Take your attention off the subject and just breathe. This will help you get your mind temporarily off the exasperation and regroup with a clearer head.

SILENT BREATHING

There is something to be said about breathing quietly – no one will hear you, even you.

This is particularly challenging if you are taking deep breaths or diaphragmatic breaths. To be silent, you pretty much need to go slowly. It is on the inhale that it might be difficult, if you have taken a full exhale with a diaphragmatic breath and you are in a desperate need for air. Reversing and trying to take in that next inhale quietly is very difficult, but doable.

Silent breathing can be matched up with any kind of breathing, really. It just takes patience and focus. It, too, helps you to slow down and be present in the moment.

RESISTANCE BREATHING

Resistance breathing is when you consciously partially block the path of breath on either your inhale or your exhale or both. By restricting your air passage in some way, you once again stimulate the respiratory system and strengthen the muscles used while you breathe.

There are lots of ways to add some resistance to your inhales and exhales. For example, you could purse your lips, breathe through a straw, breathe through a piece of cloth, clench your teeth and breathe through your mouth, or do yoga's ujjayi breathing where you tighten the back of your throat and breathe through your nose.

As with most breathing techniques, as you focus on it, you help your body relax and de-stress.

BREATHING WITH SOUND

Speaking is part of our daily behavior and we really don't think much about what happens when we speak. And, because it is a means of communication, it is the communication that is the goal, not the sound of the speech. If, however, we make the sound the priority and combine that with breathing, "magic" happens!

It's really pretty logical. The body is approximately 60% water, some say 65%, and that fluid is spread throughout the body. Sound travels incredibly well through water because of the vibration it entails. So, when you make sound while you breathe and focus on that sound, you are giving your body a bath of vibration. This bath of vibration helps soothe the parasympathetic nervous system – the half of the nervous system which controls how we feel and helps to heal us and relax us.

You can explore different chants which are directly related to what you want to focus on, or you can simply make different sounds. The well-known chant of "om" is an easy one to remember and is believed to help connect your soul to the Universe. According to several religions, the world started with one sound, and that sound was "om."

Another simple sound to make involves using the long vowel sounds of the alphabet. Inhale deeply through the nose and with your s-l-o-w exhale, make the long "a" sound: "aye." Finish your exhale sound, inhale through the nose then s-l-o-w-l-y exhale "eee." Then go through the remaining vowels, and repeat as many times as you like. You might find this very calming and invigorating at the same time.

Breathing with sound obviously makes some noise, so you do want to be respectful of those around you. Blocking your ears adds to the vibration sensation, so when you really get into it and are deeply ensconced in the sounds you are making and the breathing you are doing, you are not really thinking about imposing on other people, so consider this a fair warning – speaking from experience!

I could continue on with pages of different breathing techniques and their benefits, but I encourage you to do your own research to see what feels right for you. There are seminars and webinars and on-line classes and meditations and lectures all about different ways to breathe. What they mostly have in common are the benefits to practicing some sort of breathing exercises: reducing stress, regulating heart beats, lowering blood pressure, relieving anxiety, helping with asthma and allergies, better sleep and relief from sleep apnea and snoring. More obscurely, it has been said to help with weight loss, giving up smoking, constipation, menopause discomfort, foggy brain, and numerous other aging issues. Based on the potential for all these positive changes, I strongly recommend you find a way to incorporate some form of breathing exercise into your day. While you meditate is certainly the easiest.

Books on the subject that I recommend are:

> Breath – The New Science of a Lost Art – James Nestor
> Anatomy of Breathing – Blandine Calais-Germain
> Breath In Breathe Out – James E. Loehr, EdD and Jeffrey A. Migdow, MD
> The Healing Power of the Breath – Richard P. Brown, MD and Patricia L. Gerbarg, MD
> The Tao of Natural Breathing – Dennis Lewis

CHAPTER 6 RECAP

1) It is time to pay attention to the least expensive way to reduce stress; one that is readily available to you 24 hours a day, 7 days a week.
2) There are lots of different ways to use your breath to better your health, including nasal breathing, diaphragmatic breathing, slow breathing, silent breathing, resistance breathing, breathing with sound and hundreds of others.
3) Nasal breathing is more beneficial to the body than mouth breathing.
4) All therapeutic breathing techniques are intended to relax your parasympathetic nervous system which will, in turn, help to relieve stress as well as help with a multitude of other illnesses.
5) It's best to do your own research to find the breathing technique that is right for you.

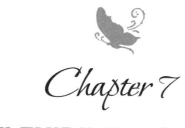

Chapter 7

FLEXIBILITY IS THE KEY TO MOBILITY

"If I knew I was going to live this long, I would have taken better care of myself."

Attributed to Mickey Mantle and others

Why don't people stretch?

What is it about stretching that people don't seem to want to include it as an important component to overall healthy exercise? No matter what the activity or sport, once the task is done or the game is over, it's on to the next thing to do. Meanwhile, our poor over-used body physically cringes because it is crying for the attention it so desperately needs.

Why don't people stretch?

I have done some polling on this and learned the reasons are few in number and almost identical. Here is what came back:

- I don't have the time
- I'll do it later (and, of course, I never get to it)
- I didn't work that hard, so it is not necessary … and my favorite:

- I know it's good for me, but I just don't do it!!

It makes me wonder, if people really understood the long-term effects of *not* stretching, would they still *not stretch*?

STRETCHING VS. WARMING UP

Through my 20+ years of fitness, I have observed that the benefits of stretching before exercising is kind of a myth. The industry has done countless studies which usually conclude that there is no real benefit to stretching before you exercise. The statistics on injury with stretching vs. not stretching before you start to exercise show pretty much that there is no advantage.

For years, diligent exercisers, bicyclists, runners and sports men and women have thought that stretching before they begin to do activities is beneficial to the body. That simply is not the case. In my opinion, stretching before you do anything is actually a bad idea, unless those muscles and joints have been warmed up.

Yes, *warming up* before getting into the strenuous part of your activity is a good thing. Proper warming up gets your blood flowing into the muscles and joints that you will be using during your exercise. It can also enhance your range of motion while you exercise.

This is important: Muscles need to be warmed up and supple *before* you stretch them. Stretching cold muscles can be dangerous because the muscle tissue can be stiff and not pliable. Engaging in stretching means literally extending the length of the muscle. If you do this with a muscle that has not been warmed up, you can potentially tear your muscle tissue or weaken it enough to instigate a tear in the future.

The easiest warmup consists of a lighter version of the activity you're about to perform. Do that for several minutes, then continue a little bit harder for a little bit longer. Total warm up time? Ten minutes is a good number. Then "play ball!"

Remember, there is no real proof that stretching before you exercise reduces the risk of injury. *Warming up* before exercising is important, but stretching? Not so much. And since *time* seems to be an issue with many people, eliminating pre-exercise stretching helps alleviate that excuse.

If you still want to stretch before you exercise, make sure you warm up for 10 minutes with the exercise you are about to perform, then do some stretching. If you are going to be playing some tennis, gently warm up with a partner for 10 minutes, then both of you stop and stretch for a few minutes, then game on! If you are going for a bike ride, ride slowly for ten minutes, then stop and stretch then continue your ride.

But you definitely want to stretch *afterwards!* Warm up *before* exercising and stretch *after* exercising – that's the protocol to follow.

STRETCHING WITH EXERCISE - WHAT TO DO AND HOW TO DO IT

As just mentioned, there is no real benefit to stretching before you exercise. But stretching afterwards is a must!

Let's think about aerobic exercise or sports. You need to warm up – get your muscles supple – before exercise to prepare your body for the exercise. Then, when your session is complete, you need to "cool down" and wait for your heart to calm down to a resting heart rate before doing your stretching. (See more about your resting heart rate in Chapter 8, *The Forgotten Muscle.*) The easiest way to do this is to simply walk around for a couple of minutes to get your heart rate back to a calmer pace after your bike ride (or your run, or your dancing – whatever your exercise choice). Or, just as you did with your warmup, do the activity at a slower pace until your heart rate comes down. This is true for stretching while standing, but even more important when lying down while you stretch. Here you want to make sure that the heart rate is calmer and at a slower resting rate to avoid any pooling of the fast-pumping blood in your heart.

Remember, we're talking here about stretching after aerobic or other strenuous activity that might elevate your heart rate. When you are strength training, your heart rate usually doesn't beat at a high aerobic rate, so you don't really need to cool down before stretching. In fact, in my BodSpir® classes, we stretch the muscle tissue right after exercising that muscle group.

The important thing for whatever stretching you do is to stay with a static stretch - put your muscle in the stretched position and hold it there for 30 seconds. Yes, I said 30 seconds. You might have heard that that much time is not necessary, but to avoid potential pain or soreness, a full 30 seconds is recommended. Again, respect what you just put your body through. Respect that your body just went full out in allowing you to do whatever exercise you chose. You should take this time and give something back to your body in gratitude for all it just did for you. Consider stretching as the best way to thank your body.

Also, a little hint to help when you go into each stretch: exhale! While you are positioning the part of the body you are stretching, before you hold it in that static position, as you ease into the stretch, exhale. That will help to relax the muscle tissue allowing you to get as much range of motion out of the stretch as you can.

There are several other kinds of stretching techniques. For instance, **ballistic stretching** incorporates a bouncing movement, often used by ballerinas to lengthen the tissue but not recommended for the kind of post-exercise stretching we are discussing, especially if unsupervised. **Dynamic stretching** is often used for warming up versus post-exercise, as it is movement that puts joints through their ranges of motion. **Passive stretching** could be done after a workout with 30-second holds, but requires an outside force (equipment) or a person assisting with putting your limbs in the stretched position.

There are quite a few other stretching techniques; however, in my experience teaching thousands of exercise classes, the static stretching technique is the most efficient. It does what you need it to do for the benefit of maintaining flexible muscle tissue. Any other technique is not necessary and really not advised unless you are doing it under the direct supervision of a trainer. You can do some serious damage, including tearing your muscle tissue, if those techniques are done incorrectly.

LET'S BE PRACTICAL

I want you to understand what you are actually doing when you stretch after exercising. When you exercise, no matter what type of exercise you choose, you continuously contract and release your muscles in order to perform the movement you need your muscles to make. This continuous contracting tends to bind up the muscle tissue, making it all gnarly and tightened together. When you take the time to stretch, you are pulling your muscles straight, elongating them, with the goal of realigning the tissue to get it back where it started from. Without stretching, your muscles stay gnarly, possibly until your next exercise session. When you do this over and over again, you eventually find that your back hurts or you can't straighten your knees or you are round-shouldered or your hip hurts…. You feel stiff. Exercise is supposed to avoid that, isn't it? I know some of you know firsthand what I am talking about.

Most forms of exercise incorporate the legs. Therefore, whatever leg stretches you do, you want to get all four quadrants of the leg: front of the thigh (quadriceps), back of the thigh (hamstrings), inner thigh (adductors) and outer thigh (abductors.) Also, stretch your calf, shin and buttocks muscles, and maybe even do some ankle circles, as all of them are involved in your exercise as well.

Pretty much all sports also involve your upper body, although it doesn't always look that way. Even with running, your posture is very important – the position of the arms, head and shoulders and how tipped forward you are. I am sure many runners could tell you of the injury or stress they have felt after a run somewhere in the upper body and not the legs. (I remember dating a bicyclist years ago who had thighs of steel and *never* worked out his upper body. He had terrible neck and lower back issues as he did not think it was important to keep those body parts strong for bike riding. After all, bike riding was all legs – right? *Wrong!*) Don't forget, the upper back, shoulders and arms should also be stretched so the muscle tissue can realign itself for repair from the strenuous activity it just performed.

Another thing you can do which will benefit your overall health is to stay quiet while stretching. Concentrate on what you are doing, focus on the muscle tissue you are stretching. Exhale as you go into the stretch and simply breathe…and hold…and breathe…and hold…for the full 30 seconds. Count "one 1,000, two 1,000," etc., so you focus on the stretching and the counting, which keeps the brain from wandering. Then move on to the next stretch. This way you are creating an intimate environment as you kindly give these rehabilitative stretches to your body to help it recuperate from the previous activity. Stretching is a gift you give back to your body in recognition of and gratitude for its ever-readiness. By adopting this inspiring attitude toward stretching, you will come to appreciate the extra time it takes and willingly incorporate it into your workout routine.

STIFFNESS IS NOT JUST IN YOUR MUSCLES

When your muscles are stiff and tight, which I am positive you have experienced, they will not only cause you pain, but will pull on your tendons. Your tendons connect your muscle tissue to your bones and your joints. So when your joints are stiff and tight, it means the tendons are pulling because the muscles are tight. *It is all connected!*

Your ligaments, which connect bone to bone, can also get tight. However, when your body is more flexible overall, the ligaments tend to perform with more flexibility as well. As with all connective tissue, staying hydrated is a key contributor to more flexibility. Tight ligaments can be very dangerous as they can tear, and if you have experienced the pain of a torn ligament, you know what I mean. A torn ligament can also take months to heal and completely disrupt your life.

The latest buzz is all about your fascia. Fascia mainly consists of tightly compacted collagen fibers that are wrapped around muscle tissue, bones, organs and blood vessels throughout your body, encasing them in a protective layer of fiber. Think of it as giant protective coverings surrounding all your moving parts on the entire inside of your body. This tissue can also get stiff and tight – mainly due to lack of movement (like sitting at a desk all day), chronic stress (something with which many working parents and/or caregivers are very familiar), dehydration, poor posture…the list goes on. Until fairly recently, fascia was pretty much ignored by the medical community. But as new information is forthcoming, we are realizing the scope of the fantastic network our body has designed to protect us. The system of fascia throughout your body allows for your insides to be individually packaged and protected, yet interconnected. It is truly an astonishing network of slippery stuff! But fascia can get tight and stiff too. In reading this chapter, as a matter of fact, you can simply add the word fascia every time you read the word muscle, as they pretty much go hand in hand.

DO YOU HAVE "JOCK KNEE"?

Many folks who exercise now were athletes in high school and college. Way back in those days – in the 60s and 70s anyway – there was very little done in the way of stretching, and if there were some stretching done, it typically occurred *before* the exercising, not after. I have worked with many former athletes, both men and women, now in their 50s and 60s, even 70s. I can honestly say every single one of them had a flexibility issue. Their biggest problem is that they cannot straighten their knees. I have even coined a phrase for this condition. I call it "jock knee"!

Want to see if you have jock knee? Sit on the floor with your back against the wall. Push your buttocks back as far as you can possibly go with your legs out in front of you. Sit up straight against the wall, with your shoulders back against the wall. Now, straighten your legs. The backs of your knees should be able to touch the floor with your toes straight up in the air - *without sliding your buttocks forward at all.*

Well? Do your knees come up off the floor more than a half-inch or so? If so, you have jock knee. How many years have you had it? Most likely it started around the time you decided to do sports and become physically active on a regular basis. Or, you were not athletic, but may spend too much time sitting or driving in a car in a seated position. And now that you are getting older, believe me it will not get better unless you do something about it. The ramifications of jock knee over time can lead to all sorts of aches and pains, especially in your posture and lower back.

There is one easy, helpful aid for jock knee that I can recommend, but keep in mind, as we have not met and I have not observed you personally, you will be doing this totally at your own risk. If the tightness behind your knees is really bad, you should check with a physiatrist (a doctor specializing in muscles and joints) or a physical therapist before doing this. As previously mentioned, the best time to do this stretch is when the muscles and connective tissue are "warmed up."

Sit up straight in a dining room chair. Push your buttocks back as far as you possibly can (just like you did on the floor). Have another dining room chair facing you with the seat open to you. Put both of your legs and feet up on it. Straighten your legs as best you can. Position your knees over the space between the seats of the two chairs. Just sit allowing the knees to relax in that openness. Depending on your situation, you could do this for anywhere from 10 seconds to 2 minutes. Judge the duration by your level of pain. If this is truly painful, even 5 seconds could be enough. Try to do it every day, once a day at first, then build to twice a day. Add a few seconds as you become more tolerant, based on your level of discomfort. Remember how many years it took for your knees to get this way. As with most successful endeavors, diligence will be the key to helping you get over your jock knee.

"SIT UP STRAIGHT!"

Another huge flexibility problem that affects millions of people is poor posture, or how we hold our bodies in space. Ever since I was a little girl,

FLEXIBILITY IS THE KEY TO MOBILITY

I remember my father reciting his boring refrain at the dinner table, "sit up straight!" Little did I know how right he was to drill me in that short command. To this day, I have always monitored my posture and can proudly say that I have never had an issue with it. There are many, however, who did not grow up as lucky as I did in that regard.

The most common issue that arises from poor posture is rounded shoulders, which, over time, results in all sorts of physical problems – problems that vary with each afflicted person. Plus, it is simply not an attractive feature at any age. How is your posture? Want to check? The following activity has enlightened – and in some cases, stunned – many, many people as to exactly how "off" their posture might be. (Again, you are doing this activity completely at your own risk, recognizing that there is a possibility of imbalance.)

Stand against a wall facing out, with your heels against the baseboard and your feet hip-width apart and parallel. Stand up straight and put your shoulders back as far as you can, pressing against the wall. Your head should be able to touch the wall *without* tilting it back. If your head doesn't hit the wall, simply make sure that your shoulders are back and that *your chin is level and parallel with the floor.* Look straight ahead. Arms are by your sides with palms facing in toward the sides of your thighs. You with me? Now, just stand there for about 15 to 20 seconds. Keep the shoulders back and the chin level.

When you are ready, *do not move anything* except your legs: Take one step away from the wall, bring the other foot forward, and stand still. Shoulders should still be back, chin level, arms by your sides, feet parallel. The big question: How does that feel? I'll bet that for 99 out of 100 people, it feels incredibly awkward. You are now standing in your version of "perfect posture." Theoretically, this is how you should be walking and standing all the time. What do you think? How weird does it feel for you? Time to pay attention? Want to remedy your posture?

To help you restore your posture, simply do this activity every day, two or three times a day, standing in "perfect posture" for about 30 seconds. Over time – and I mean a long time (again, think of how long it took you to get out of perfect posture) – slowly but surely, you might be able to recapture that straighter stance. Remember, your muscles have memory - they can recall how you used to stand and, in time, they will try to get you back to that. But it is your daily diligence in retraining the muscles that will lead you to success.

MUSCLE MEMORY - DO YOUR MUSCLES REALLY REMEMBER?

In a word, yes, they do! Without getting too scientific, there is a pathway between the brain and your muscle tissue. When a particular exercise activity is performed over and over again, the connection is imbedded in the brain and a blueprint, of sorts, gets filed away. So, if you stop the activity, even for years, it is much easier for you to get back into it than for someone who is new at the endeavor. Your muscle memory, that blueprint, resurfaces so that the activity is easier to perform. This has been proven in study after study with mice as well as humans.

Why is that important for stretching and flexibility? The body knows the stasis position it is supposed to be in. I am sure at some point in your life, your body knew how to stand up straight. Since then, if the muscles in your shoulders have over-stretched in your upper back and tightened up in your chest and you are now round-shouldered, you can work at regaining your former perfect posture with time and lots of practice. And, depending on the severity of your poor posture, you may need to do additional exercises and stretches to help offset the years of rounding. (As I do not know your specific issue, I must qualify here and say that this is possible in most scenarios, but every case is, in fact, different.)

One more word about posture. If you found your "perfect posture" to be less than perfect, and you do not start trying to fix it, *it will not get any better than it is right now. It will only get worse!* And poor posture can lead to back pain, shoulder pain, neck pain and rounded shoulders, which can crowd the ribs and make it harder to breathe. Poor posture can also give rise to a poor gait, which can cause problems in the hips, knees and ankles. The list goes on. Poor posture is a very strong indication of how your body will age and, therefore, how you will age. So, if it's not worth a few minutes a day to reprogram your body to "sit up straight" now, don't be surprised when you become a bent over little old lady or man!

The key to flexibility and mobility is practice, practice, practice. If you want to enhance your flexibility in any way, you *must* stretch over and over again, day after day after day, in order to regain any flexibility that you have lost over the decades.

"I've never been able to touch my toes!" I can't count how many times I have heard that. The thing is, our bodies are made in such proportion that we should be able to touch our toes. People who can touch their toes are not *overly* flexible, they are the way they should be.

Again, I'm going to suggest some activities which, if you choose to do them, are at your own risk. Bend over, *without bending your knees*, and try to touch the floor. The number of inches your fingertips are off the floor can be a measurement of your flexibility.

If you are carrying too much weight in your girth, this little test will not be a true reading of your flexibility. The following strap exercise, however, will be. Lie on your back with your knees bent. Put a strap (an old tie or a belt will do) underneath the ball of the *right* foot. Straighten the right leg completely, holding onto the strap with both hands. When the right knee is straight, gently lift that leg up into the air as high as you can *without bending the knee*. (There is a danger in hyperextending the knee, which is pushing the kneecap too far back into the joint. To avoid this, be sure to straighten the knee without overdoing it.) Ideally, your leg should be at a 90° angle from the floor, i.e., straight up in the air. As I said, this is ideal. If, however, your leg is only 75° from the floor, you have some work to do!

If you already have self-diagnosed "jock knee," that will certainly contribute to an angle less than 90°. Use the jock knee stretch using two chairs described above to help alleviate that problem. However, if you don't have jock knee and you still have less than a 90° angle to the floor, repeat this floor stretch once or twice a day and hold it for 30 to 60 seconds. As with all stretches, that may be difficult at first. Start out at only 5 to 10 seconds and slowly build up to a longer period of time. *Make sure that you are warmed up first!*

Remember, your muscles remember where they belong and how they should be positioned in relation to each other. If your behavior over the years has taken them outside their ideal location or extension, they will do the best they can to get back to where they should be. But they can't do anything without your help and initiation of the stretch.

THE BOTTOM LINE ON STRETCHING

So, let's get to the bottom line on why stretching is so important. The #1 reason to stretch is to avoid being stiff. Not just stiff today or tomorrow, but next week, next month, next year, even next decade.

If you decide that you just don't have time to stretch, I can guarantee that your body will slowly but surely begin to tighten up and shrink up. And, before you know it, you won't be able to stand up straight. You won't be able to get in and out of the car easily. You won't be able to get up and down off the couch easily. And worst of all, you will become that bent-over little old lady (or man) you swore you would never become.

The key to avoiding this, and to taking control of your aging with agility and flexibility, is to stretch every day. Not just after your exercise of choice. I urge you to begin a regular stretching routine of your own each and every day. There are countless people waking up with their "Warming Up With BodSpir®" recording each morning, taking 20 minutes to warm up their bodies for the day ahead. You should try it! Your body will thank you by giving back all day long!!

THE BOTTOM LINE ON NOT STRETCHING

So, here's a question: What aging issue is most affected by having stiff muscles and joints? I really want you to take a moment to think about this. If you are having trouble moving because various muscle tissue is inflexible, how would that affect your overall functionality? If you can't move as easily as you would like to because you have so much stiffness, how is that going to affect your life?

Chances are, what will be affected the most as you age is your balance. If you accidently trip while walking, your reaction time plays a role, but if your brain quickly registers the trip and the muscles are activated to avoid the fall, will your muscles be supple enough to react?

Fear of falling is terrifying for the elderly, and for good reason. "Falls are the leading cause of injury among adults aged ≥65 years (older adults) in the United States. In 2018, an estimated 3 million emergency department visits, more than 950,000 hospitalizations or transfers to another facility (e.g., trauma center), and approximately 32,000 deaths resulted from fall-related injuries among older adults."[30]

Although I appreciate the fact that you may not be elderly now, and this issue is 10 to 30 years in the future for you, it's never too soon to pay attention. You certainly don't want to fall at the age of 75 and have it affect the rest of your life, and the life of your family.

Certainly, there are other factors involved with falling aside from lack of flexibility. A few are muscle weakness, a sedentary lifestyle, problems with your gait or trouble with balance. Muscle weakness can be helped through strength training. A sedentary lifestyle can be helped by getting up and moving. Issues with your gait are generally caused by a lack of strength, inflexibility and poor balance. However, it can often develop due to some injury in the lower body causing one to walk differently to offset pain. People with a gait issue need to seek help from physical therapy to focus on normalizing their walking pattern. If they choose not to pay attention, their future mobility is in jeopardy.

---

[30] nih.org (National Institutes of Health), National Library of Medicine, "Trends in Nonfatal Falls and Fall-Related Injuries Among Adults Aged ≥ 65 Years - United States, 2012-2018"

As for balance, there is a lot you can do. Staying in balance has to do with proprioception (also known as kinesthesia) and the body's ability to sense your movement and where you are located in space. It is inherent in your muscle tissue with every movement you make. Your proprioceptive system needs to be functioning normally in order for you to keep your balance. Paying attention to this sensory information you receive from your skin, nerves in the feet and the muscles and connective tissue in your ankles and feet also help with balance. Your awareness of your surroundings *all the time* helps you stay in balance. Maintaining good posture also helps to keep control of your balance.

Keep in mind that balance problems can be caused by issues in your inner ear which manifest in dizziness or disorientation, which, in turn, can cause imbalance. Poor eyesight can also be a factor, keeping you from seeing those hidden hazards in your path. Be aware of potential side effects of any medications, as some may impair your balance. How quickly you can react to a stumble is very important and has everything to do with your flexibility and focus – things you can work to control!

To determine if you may have an issue with balance do this very simple test. (Reminder that you are doing this completely at your own risk.) Stand up straight with your feet together, shoulders back and chin level as best you can. If you can stand steadily without swaying, that is a good thing. If you are not swaying, try closing your eyes. If you sway in either case, you need to start working on your balance. If you are able to stay steady without swaying, chances are your balance is good for now, but you still need to make sure you are doing all the right things to maintain it.

FLEXIBILITY IS THE KEY TO MOBILITY

Think about everything you have done so far today up to sitting down and reading this book, this chapter, this line. Did you notice any stiffness at all today? Did you have any trouble walking at all today? Getting up from a chair? The floor? Did you get in and out of the car? Was it easy? Did you pick something up off the floor? How was it straightening back up? All these activities and the hundreds more you have performed today were affected by your flexibility, or lack thereof. If all is well and there were no issues, keep up the good work. But keep in mind, how you felt today is the best you will feel for the rest of your life – your mobility will deteriorate with age – unless you proactively work to maintain or improve it. Your body cannot do it without you.

CHAPTER 7 RECAP

1) Stretching before you exercise does not help offset injury.
2) Warming up before exercise is the best way to prepare your muscles for what is to come.
3) Stretching after exercise is the best way to realign your muscle tissue.
4) Stiff muscles are just the tip of the iceberg. Stiffness in your fascia, tendons and ligaments also affects your flexibility.
5) The inability to straighten the back of the knee can eventually lead to poor posture and lower back issues.
6) Poor posture can lead to a myriad of problems as you age.
7) Muscle memory is a real thing and can be retrieved even if lost for decades, though it will take time.
8) Incorporating stretching into your daily routine is the best way to avoid stiffness as time goes by. This stiffness is a great contributor to balance problems as we age.
9) Stiffness and poor balance contribute to the huge fear of falling that develops as we get older.
10) Flexibility is truly the key to mobility.

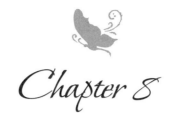

Chapter 8

THE FORGOTTEN MUSCLE

> *"Life is like riding a bicycle. To keep your balance, you must keep moving."*
>
> *Albert Einstein*

Certainly, you have heard that some thoughts "come from your heart and not your head." When we point at ourselves, we point directly to our hearts. Valentine's Day cards and celebrations are filled with hearts. How did the heart become the symbol for love? And how did the heart become the symbol for our emotional center?

The heart is, indeed, a unique organ. We need the heart to pump blood throughout the body. Blood carries oxygen and nutrients to our various organs and tissues so that they, too, may survive and thrive. It is the one organ that is physically connected to all the others because of this flow of blood. When the heart is malnourished or sickly, it cannot function at its peak potential. And, as we all know, when the heart stops functioning, oxygen cannot get to the brain and we die. Interestingly, it is the heart's last beat that determines our death, not the cessation of the brain's function.

In the United States there are far too many sick hearts. Statistics from the Center for Disease Control tell us that:[31]

---

[31] cdc.gov/heartdisease/facts, "Heart Disease in the United States"

- Heart disease is the leading cause of death for both men and women.
- In 2020, one in five deaths was from some form of heart disease.
- In the United States alone, someone has a heart attack every 40 seconds.
- Every 34 seconds, one person in the United States dies from some form of cardiovascular disease.

The saddest part of these staggering numbers is that most heart-related events are preventable. That's right - preventable. So, if heart disease is mostly preventable, why is it the number one killer of men and women?

Heart diseases have been linked to a growing epidemic, not only here in the US but throughout the world: Obesity. We literally are what we eat, and what we are eating is simply not good for us. Therefore, to dramatically reduce the odds of a heart disease diagnosis, you need to maintain a reasonable weight for your height. Eating smart is an entire book in itself, but if you are looking to start making changes, eat more vegetables and less sugar. Cut out the simple carbohydrates (white flour foods). Reduce your meat consumption and include fish as a protein. (See more in Chapter 9, *You Are What You Eat.*) The options are readily available for you to make healthier choices. It is up to you to make the commitment to select and implement those choices.

A LITTLE MORE ABOUT THE HEART AND YOUR DIET

I am not a heart expert, nor am I a dietician. I do, however, hold a Specialty Certification in Fitness Nutrition. More importantly, I know where to go to learn and get the best information about diet and the heart. What I just said is a good start: Eat more vegetables and less sugar. Reduce your meat consumption and include fish as a protein. Avoid fried foods and saturated fats.

To explore this in more detail, visit Dr. Dean Ornish at www.ornish.com. Dr. Ornish has a program directly related to preventing or reversing heart disease while promoting overall good health.

There is a plethora of heart healthy programs relating to diet that are available to the public. If you currently have a healthy heart, you most likely do not have a cardiologist. So, speak to your primary care physician and see if they have any recommended programs you could research. Or, better still, do your own research and find the program that works for you. Then talk to your doctor. Discuss what you have found out and see what he or she recommends for you.

The bottom line is clear. If you want a healthy heart, you must have a healthy diet. Since we know 80% of cardiovascular disease is preventable,[32] wouldn't you want to make the right choices? Not just for you, but for your family?

THE HEART/BRAIN CONNECTION

What we see with our eyes transmits to the brain to translate what it is we are looking at. What we hear with our ears does the same thing. Our senses of touch, taste and smell all work that way as well. Our senses do their jobs, communicate to the brain and we then understand what we need to about the stimulus. When our senses sense, there is a series of neurological transmissions that occur to facilitate our knowing about that information. The same goes for the heart.

According to Dr. J. Andrew Armour in his 1991 book Neurocardiology, the heart has its own "little brain." This "heart brain" is composed of approximately 40,000 neurons that are like the neurons in the brain, meaning that the heart has its own nervous system.

In addition, the heart communicates with the brain in four major ways: neurologically (through the transmission of nerve impulses), biochemically (via hormones and neurotransmitters), biophysically (through pressure waves) and energetically (through electromagnetic field interactions). Communication along all these conduits significantly affects the brain's activity.[33]

---

[32] heart.org (American Heart Association), "CDC Prevention Programs"
[33] Science of the Heart: Exploring the Role of the Heart in Human Performance, Heartmath Institute, 2019

Afferent, or sensory, nerves are responsible for bringing sensory information from the outside world to the brain. The vagus nerve, which is 80% afferent, carries information from the heart and other internal organs to the brain. Signals from the "heart brain" redirect to the medulla, hypothalamus, thalamus, and amygdala and the cerebral cortex. Thus, the heart sends more signals to the brain than vice versa.[34]

What this means is that our emotions communicate with the brain which communicates with the heart. When we are overwrought or stressed or sad or depressed or angry, our brain and heart communicate back and forth, each reacting with their own physiological response. The brain is having its strong physiological reaction to the situation, but so is the heart. The combination of the two could literally give you a heart attack from a highly stressful situation or emotion.

The good news is that we can help ourselves, in the heat of the moment. If you feel your emotions are becoming piqued and not in a good way, along with taking a few deep breaths, try to think of good things and situations and people that you love and care for. If you are a passionate skier, imagine yourself at your favorite slope, schussing down. If you love nature, envision a woodlands or meadow where your favorite creatures appear. Maybe it's your children or grandchildren – picture them in your mind. It is very important to actually sense the emotion that you would feel when you are with a particular person or in a specific situation. If you can get off the negativity of the heated emotion and focus on things in your life that make you feel good, go there. Continue your slow deep breathing, ideally through the nose until you get a sense of relief.

You really do have the tools you need to help support your heart and your brain through whatever emotions you are feeling. When they are good, go with it and put a smile on your face. And, when they are not good, focus on turning them around. It is so much better for your heart, your body and your overall health.

---

[34] nih.gov (National Institutes of Health), National Library of Medicine, "Pain: Is It All in the Brain or the Heart?" 2019

THE HEART IS A MUSCLE

An important fact we often forget is that the heart is a muscle. As with all muscles, it needs to be exercised to be strong and stay strong.

We lose a half-pound of muscle tissue every year beginning in our early 30s. And because the heart is a muscle, it does undergo some atrophy as we age.

Under the best circumstances, assuming your body is at its proper healthy weight, the heart pumps approximately 100,000+ times per day, circulating about 2,000 gallons of blood per day, or 5-6 quarts per minute. That is a lot of work! The heart needs to be strengthened so that it can keep up with all this pumping. When you are even just 10 pounds overweight, your heart must work harder to accommodate the additional demand. If you are more than 35 pounds overweight, there is a dramatic amount of stress added to the level of exertion, even with normal everyday tasks. So, one way to maintain a healthy heart is to maintain a healthy weight.

Another consideration when you are overweight, especially if you are more than 35 pounds overweight, is to take into account where the extra fat that you are carrying is located. There are basically two kinds of fat: visceral fat, which is inside your body wrapped around your organs, and subcutaneous fat, which is what we more easily see – the fat stored below the skin.

It is the visceral fat we need to worry about when it comes to your heart. Even an extra ounce or two of fat physically surrounding your heart (pericardial fat, a type of visceral fat) forces your heart to work even harder to pump 100,000+ times a day. That is a lot of extra exertion from one muscle.

An aerobics program, along with strength training, will certainly help you lose any extra weight. However, it is very important that you respect your body's current condition and go slowly in beginning your aerobics program. Allow a gradual increase in intensity based on the signals your body gives you and let that be your guide on how slowly or quickly you progress. Do not go full out, as that can put too much stress on your heart muscle, but build up to it and let your body and heart be by your side rather than always trying to catch up.

The best way to do that is to include aerobic exercise as part of your exercise regimen on a *regular* basis and welcome it as a part of your daily life. Just be sure to start at a lower intensity and gradually build up your heart's capacity to pump blood and oxygen to the rest of your body.

AEROBIC EXERCISE - EXERCISE "IN OXYGEN"

Aerobic exercise is the best way to keep your heart muscle strong for decades to come. According to the American College of Sports Medicine, which sets up exercise and physical activity guidelines in the fitness industry, aerobic exercise should be done a minimum of 5 times per week, getting your heart in your own "moderate intensity aerobic zone" for a minimum of 30 continuous minutes each time. Or, for the more vigorous exerciser, 3 times per week for a minimum of 20 minutes at a faster, higher intensity.[35] If you need to lose weight, you will want to build up to a good hour each day in addition to strength training and other self-care options. That will help boost your metabolism which will help burn calories more efficiently to lose weight more easily. Most importantly, you need to find what works for you and what level of discipline you are able to uphold.

If you are just beginning, start slowly and go for shorter stretches of time. Then start increasing the duration before you increase the intensity. Be careful not to overexert when you start. Have realistic expectations and set yourself up to succeed each time you exercise. Beating yourself up with disappointment is only going to discourage you from doing it again.

Here is a great example of getting started. Take a walk. How does it feel? How long can you walk comfortably before it feels exertive and hard to do? Make note of both your times and the distance you walked. Then the next time you walk, try to go just a little bit farther. For my local clients, and this might work for you, I suggest they count telephone poles. Each

---

[35] *ACSM's Guidelines for Exercise Testing and Prescription*, 11th edition, 2021

day or few days, they increase by half to one full distance between poles. When they can walk three miles, we start increasing their time and aim to do it faster. Are you the aggressive type and want to go faster sooner? That is a choice you can make. The important thing is this: YOU know your body; YOU feel your body; only YOU can evaluate what your body is asking for and can support. By the way, tracking your activity applies to any type of aerobics. As you feel your personal endurance is increasing, it means the muscles have gotten stronger (including your heart) and you are now ready to be pushed further – always gradually.

When your muscles are working harder than normal, they call for more oxygen in order to function efficiently. The oxygen comes from the blood, so the heart will kick into gear and pick up the pace to deliver that oxygen to the demanding muscles. Everything works harder and stress is added, but in a good way.

Be cautious not to push yourself too hard, especially in the beginning. You want to push yourself past your normal level of exertion - I call this pushing past your "normalcy" - and that is all it takes. A good start is to build up to 5 times per week for 30 minutes or more. My tried and true recommendation is this: When you reach a solid routine at this level of aerobic exercise on a regular basis for a minimum of six months, then you might be ready for anaerobic exercise. I say you *might be*, because I also recommend that your doctor is aware of your exercise regimen and your exertion levels.

ANAEROBIC EXERCISE - EXERCISE "OUT OF OXYGEN"

Athletes, in their training, typically perform past their normalcy, then step it up by pushing the heart rate past its comfortable level of exertion. In other words, asking it to work up to 85% of its capacity. One form of this exercise strategy is called HIIT – High Intensity Interval Training – a form of anaerobic exercise. During a HIIT workout, your heart rate can go way up to accommodate what is being demanded, but it does so in a very short time frame. One example is to do your HIIT workout twice a week – walk 3½-4 miles per hour for 3 minutes, then run 5-6 miles per hour for one minute. Repeat this pattern for 35 minutes. That gives eight bursts of effort that push your heart into the anaerobic zone.

Important note: Being anaerobic for any period of time, by definition, means you are exercising "out of oxygen." You will not be able to maintain the pace as your muscles will not be able to get the oxygen they need and your body will simply hit a wall of exhaustion.

Many sports, such as tennis, basketball or soccer, take you into an anaerobic state temporarily with spurts of energy followed by relative calm. If it's your goal to participate in any such active sport at your peak performance level, it is best to train your heart aerobically and get it strong. When you are ready and armed with knowledge and practice, incorporating anaerobic exercise into your weekly program will certainly help you maintain a healthy and fit heart. But please don't try it if you are just beginning an exercise program.

KINDS OF AEROBIC EXERCISE

There are many types of aerobic exercise from which to choose. As mentioned, walking is a great way to start. You just have to make sure that your pace is giving you enough of a workout and that your heart is pumping in your preferred range. Pumping your arms or using walking sticks helps.

I do not recommend running unless you are at a perfect body weight. You should begin by walking fast and getting your body into the mechanics of running before you move into the actual motion of running. Injury can happen too easily when you run, especially if your body isn't ready for it.

Honestly, I never recommend running for anyone! I have had way too many clients who were injured from running in their earlier years. I see the aftermath of it and it is not good. Our bodies were simply not made for that degree of pounding on our knees and hips, never mind feet and ankles. I know a handful of people who have been running for decades, and every one of them has had physical issues with one joint or the other related to running. It is my opinion there are many other forms of aerobics available that are far less abusive to our bodies.

The key to being successful with aerobic exercise is finding something that you enjoy doing. Because if you do not enjoy doing it, you simply won't do it. I started taking aerobics classes at a gym over 30 years ago when I had just had my second child. I was 50 pounds overweight and I knew that we wanted at least one more child. I wasn't about to get pregnant until I lost weight! I really enjoyed the classes and the challenge of the choreography. Plus, the instructor was lots of fun. Today I prefer step aerobics for all the same reasons and do DVDs in my studio. It entertains me while challenging me, so I am diligent with it and stick to a regular schedule.

No matter which form of aerobics you choose, you want to make sure you go through a warmup, get your heart rate into an exertive (but not overly exertive) zone and, when you are ready, keep it there for at least 30 minutes. Then allow a cool-down to get your heart rate back to normal.

Here are some of the many options you can choose from:

- Aerobics - DVDs, online, classes
- Walking - If you walk fast enough to get your heart beating faster than normal
- Bicycling - Same rules as walking. Start slowly and keep going a little further each ride. Once you are biking about 10 miles, try to speed it up and challenge your time.
- Elliptical machine - Found in most gyms, along with all other cardio machines - the reclining bike, stair climber, stationary bike and more.
- Spin classes - I recommend spinning only after you have a bit of aerobic experience. Spinning can be very challenging for the beginner and take you more into your anaerobic zone versus your aerobic zone. The instructors are very hard-driving, because most people in the class want it that way. Should you make this choice, find a spin instructor who has experience with beginners and

"older" folk. They should be flexible with how they teach the class, and remember – YOU control your heart rate.
- Swimming - A fabulous full body workout and aerobic workout at the same time. Again, start small and build up those laps or longer swims.

The goal is to find an exercise regimen that you enjoy, that you will actually do, and that allows you to control your level of exertion.

Let me be clear: The only reason you are building an aerobic exercise regimen is to exercise your heart! It's not about playing a sport or winning a game. It is about taking thirty minutes or more, five days a week, to give your heart and your body what they need, in gratitude for everything your heart and your body do for you. And, because your heart is a muscle, it, too, needs to be strengthened. It is through a smart aerobic exercise program that works for you (and that you will actually do) that you can maintain a stronger heart.

JUST ONE MORE THING…

And I can't emphasize this enough. To be successful at aerobics, you want to avoid injury. The best way to avoid injury is to make sure that your legs are strong enough for the aerobic exercise you are doing. So, strengthen those thighs as discussed in the BodSpir® chapter, and support your heart and the rest of your body by giving your legs the strength they need to support the demands you are making. If that means waiting a month or two while you begin your strength training program to get those legs stronger, so be it. As I have said many times, if this is the rest of your life, you have plenty of time.

CHAPTER 8 RECAP

1) There is a very strong relationship between the heart and the brain.
2) The heart is responsible for pumping the blood throughout your body, which carries the oxygen that all organs and tissue need to function.
3) As with all muscles, the heart is subject to atrophy with age.
4) Aerobic exercise is exercise "in oxygen" and comes in a variety of choices: aerobics classes or videos, walking (provided you walk fast enough to increase your heart rate) bicycling, elliptical machine, stair climber, stationary bike, spin classes (approach with caution!) and swimming, to name a few.
5) The safest way to do aerobics is to keep your legs strong to accommodate the demands you are making on them when doing the exercise.

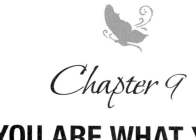

Chapter 9
YOU ARE WHAT YOU EAT – LITERALLY!

"Let food be thy medicine, let medicine be thy food."

Hippocrates

Eating healthy food has become complicated and inconvenient, and most agree it is also costly. Consequently, most don't do it. I mean, who has the time, the patience or the pocketbook, right?

It is my hope that after you read this chapter, you will see why it is important to pay attention to the facts and to start your journey of eating more healthfully. There is a very valid health reason for investing your time, your effort and energy, and yes, your money. What I am presenting to you here is really just the tip of the iceberg for healthy eating, but it is comprehensive enough to make a huge difference in the journey to a healthy older age.

I have been studying this for more than twenty years and sometimes feel I have barely scratched the surface. However, in sharing what I *have* learned I hope to get you excited and inspired to make changes in both food and diet. I hope this will be a wake-up call to encourage you to take a giant step forward, making a conscious decision to eat healthfully and provide for your physical future.

Please understand that I am not a scientist and I am also not a fan of overwhelming statistics. The ideas I am sharing are presented in human-speak from a non-scientific and non-analytical perspective. What I am summarizing and offering to you is not a made-up theory, but one derived from research that I have incorporated into my personal eating style and helped my clients incorporate into theirs. Realizing you might never have seen or thought about these concepts, I want to impress upon you that research backs up all my recommendations. I encourage you to take a vested interest in what you put into your body and do your own research that is specific to your needs and desires. You will be amazed at how much information you will find to support your healthy food choices.

It is important that we first take the time to learn a bit of history and the impact it has had on not just our food choices, but our overall health and physical wellness.

WHERE IT ALL BEGAN

Man, as a walking, upright being, has been around for an estimated 200,000 years.

In the beginning we ate mostly fruits, honey, plants, small animals and birds, and big meat that the "hunter" men brought home. These foods were not necessarily in the same form as those being consumed today. How our bodies digested that food and used the nutrients from it was how our bodies were meant to process food.

The evolution of the agricultural age began some 10,000 – 12,000 years ago. This was when we started to grow food and grains, tubers and other root vegetables and added them to our diet. A few thousand years after that, we started to domesticate animals and corral them for the ultimate purpose of slaughter and consumption. Most common were the likes of goats and sheep. We continued in this healthy innocence, adding more fruits and vegetables and animals. Then, as we began circumnavigating the globe, we added foods from other countries. In the United States, we progressed through the centuries until about halfway into the 20th century. It was then, sometime around the mid-1950s, when the demand for bulk-farmed food began.

The population was growing rapidly. Eventually, "supermarkets" cropped up, designed to hold larger quantities and inventories of multitudes of food varieties. It was also around this time when the government stepped in. They had a goal to help subsidize the farmers so farmers could produce more bulk products – like soy, wheat and corn, just to name a few – to feed the growing population. There was more demand on the farmer to farm more efficiently so that the store shelves could be filled regularly. Losing crops to bugs and pests was a detriment to the farmers' business. Though more natural pesticides had been used for thousands of years, more efficient toxic pesticides and ways to control crop production were developed. Enter the chemical companies and their synthetic versions of pest killers. With a goal of helping farmers, they introduced the ability to minimize crop damage by spraying pesticides, herbicides, and insecticides onto the growing crops. What is important to note here is that there was minimal, if any, testing done on the impact to the food and to the human that consumed it.

Agriculture moved into an era when farmers had the ability to increase crop sizes on an enormous scale, mostly because regular chemical spraying allowed crops to survive pest destruction.

In 1974, one of the most dangerous chemicals relating to human food consumption was released by Monsanto: Roundup, the weed killer. We are a nation that values economic growth, and while we can fall back on some innocence, we also have to admit to a blind ignorance as we trusted the "powers that be" to safeguard our wellbeing. In this case, that trust was misplaced. Roundup contains the chemical glyphosate - which is linked to so many illnesses, I cannot even provide you with a number. Health risks include cancer, liver and kidney damage, reproductive and developmental issues and much more. I do encourage you to google "glyphosate" and you will come up with over 14,000,000 links to click on to learn the history of glyphosate and the extensive damage it has done to the land and to the health of people around the globe. What is most shocking is that Roundup has been banned or restricted in 25 countries throughout the world,[36] but not in the United States. However, state governments in half of the United States have imposed restrictions on the use of this carcinogen. We are getting there!!

It is a fact that since the mid-20th century people are sicker on a day-to-day basis than we ever have been before. More and more people suffer from allergies, colds and flu, asthma, bowel issues like colitis, diverticulitis, Irritable Bowel Syndrome and Crohn's Disease. We are seeing earlier starts to the spread of brain diseases like dementia and Alzheimer's. Cancer is rampant! Neurological disorders in the form of Parkinson's disease, multiple system atrophy, multiple sclerosis, autism, kidney failure and liver disease are all on the rise.

Would it be safe to say that pretty much *every organ and system* of the human body is being attacked or compromised? The important question to ask is, were these diseases around *before* mid-century? While the answer is obviously yes, the numbers show staggering increases since then!

Please understand. I am not solely blaming the chemicals sprayed on our food for our current unhealthy human condition. However, many studies have shown that those chemicals are major players in compromising the immune system and compromising it so badly that our own body is unable to sufficiently defend itself! Ironically, our sick immune system, unable to do its job, is the reason why humans are getting sicker and sicker.

For the past 99,900 years, our digestive system was doing just fine for the most part. When we look at the past 70 years, the ingestion of these foreign substances has been so vast that there simply hasn't been enough time for our bodies to mutate into whatever form is needed to accommodate, or stave off, these poisons.

---

[36] hrw.org/news (Human Rights Watch), "United States Should Ban Use of Glyphosate on Food Crops," July 2020

PROCESSED FOODS

It is not just the chemicals that have our bodies trying to figure things out; it was during this same period that our growing population wanted more convenience. Manufacturers saw opportunity in the production of processed foods. Food manufacturers from all corners wanted to make things easier for the lady in the kitchen – ergo the explosion of boxed pancake mix, pre-made cookies, tinned vegetables, savory snacks … the list goes on and on. These packaged foods flooded the aisles of the supermarkets. "Cheese food" vs. cheese became more common and the selection of breakfast cereals doubled every few years. In making bread more commercially viable, we sacrificed the healthy nutrients, which were stripped out of the grain to be more easily manipulated and then put back into the loaves in bulk. This manipulated additive was promoted as "enriched" flour. Sounds like a good thing, but truthfully not.

By creating processed foods and pulverizing grains into a fine powder so that the bread or cereal or cracker or cookie could be made, simple carbohydrates were created from what used to be more complex carbohydrates. Carbohydrates provide our reserve of energy; the more complex, the longer lasting. By decimating the integrity of the grain, the quality of the carbohydrate was also decimated. Left over was a simpler carbohydrate that, as far as the body is concerned, is sugar. And although it doesn't taste like the sweet table sugar our tongues are used to, those simple carbohydrates are digested and processed in our bodies just like white sugar.

THE MANY FACES OF SUGAR: READ YOUR LABELS!

Because consuming simple carbohydrates is the same as eating sugar, the overriding issue with processed foods is the amount of carbohydrates that are in these foods.

The U.S. Department of Agriculture states that the average American consumes 156 pounds of sugar each year. That's 3 pounds of sugar each week, or 0.43 pounds of sugar each day! **That's 1 cup of sugar each day**

per person. Yikes! It is important for you to know where that sugar is hidden and what foods you can eliminate to help reduce your overall sugar consumption.

One problem with all this sugar is that it is highly addictive – that is why Frito-Lay was so clever in their advertising promotion with Lays Potato Chips, "Betcha can't eat just one!" They knew what they were selling – addictive sugars! Since the majority of processed food turns into sugar once we digest it, we really have a difficult time calling any of these foods nutritious.

Let me give you an example of how to determine the actual sugar content in a processed food. Here is a sample of a nutrition label from the FDA.

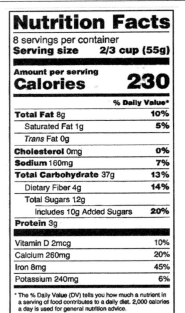

Dietary fiber is a complex carbohydrate. All other carbohydrates are simple carbohydrates, which are processed by the body as sugar. So, to calculate the amount of sugar in your food, subtract the number of grams of dietary fiber from the total number of grams of carbohydrates. In this case, 37 – 4 = 33 grams of sugar. To convert grams to teaspoons, divide the number of grams by 4.

This 8-ounce serving has over 8 teaspoons of sugar!

Notice that the manufacturer would have you believe that the amount of sugar is only 12 grams, which is equal to 3 teaspoons. That doesn't seem as bad, right? But when you actually account for all the simple carbohydrates (that is, what's left when you don't count the fiber) – the amount is disturbing.

So, next time you are grocery shopping, check out the labels and do some simple arithmetic. You will be shocked.

Now, because there is little to no nutritional value that sugar offers the body, you most likely will find yourself getting hungry just a couple of hours after consuming a meal with high sugar content. Things like pastas and breads, once digested, are treated like sugar by your body and the chemical reaction to sugar begins. Or should I say, the sugar *addiction* begins.

YOUR BODY'S CHEMICAL REACTION TO SUGAR

When sugar is ingested, there is a chemical response in the brain which releases the feel-good chemicals of serotonin and dopamine. As with feel-good narcotics, we crave more and more. And so we tend to eat more. In addition, our pancreas releases more insulin into the blood stream to help neutralize the now increased level of sugar in our blood. Remember, the body is ALWAYS driving towards a state of homeostasis and balance. So, when all of a sudden the amount of sugar we ingest is too high for normal insulin levels, our system reacts to stabilize everything. In a fairly reasonable time period, all systems are back to "normal" but the body is exhausted, so there is a sense of a "crash," and fatigue sets in. Time for a nap! Unfortunately, our body remembers the physiological reaction we had to the sugar and we want more. We want that feel-good sensation again. Especially when we are going through a rough time, we often reach for "comfort foods," which are delivering that sugar hit to us – helping us feel better emotionally. Unfortunately, the relief is temporary but the useless calories are not, and those useless calories play a more serious role in our health.

The addictive nature of sugar is obvious, so when more and more sugar was added to our food production, we were headed for serious trouble. People would naively be eating cereal or a bagel for breakfast, bread in a sandwich at lunch and pasta for dinner. Having ingested too much sugar in a day without being able to burn it off, the body stores the excess sugar as fat. And so the obesity epidemic began.

The upsurge of monitoring our cholesterol began in the 1960s. Health advisors determined that the cholesterol found in fatty foods was bad for us. As a result, the food manufacturers eliminated or reduced the fat in many foods. Unfortunately, removing the fat removed the flavor!

In order to re-enhance the flavor, they added, you guessed it, SUGAR! And not just cane sugar. Farmers were growing enormous crops of corn, so high fructose corn syrup was created, which is a higher concentrate of sugar. And again, when sugar is consumed and not burned off right away, it turns to fat. And that is what happened to the American population: WE GOT FAT!

SIZE MATTERS!

Let me begin this section with a perspective…

If you are reading this and have had a weight issue throughout your life, I really understand your difficulties. As I shared earlier, for as long I can remember, I have always weighed 10-15 pounds more than I wanted. I didn't feel worthy of a lighter body that I could wear with pride – so I kept that extra weight on. It was, in a way, my own security blanket, even though it did not make me happy.

I greatly respect that my ten pounds could be your 20, 30 or even 100 pounds. While that presents an even tougher challenge to control, it is the self-disappointment and self-loathing that is the same for all of us, no matter if it is 10 pounds or 100 pounds.

When I chose fitness as a profession, one of my biggest reasons was in knowing it would force me to get into and stay in good shape. And it has!

BUT there is something so very important I learned that relates to all of us.

What I have learned is that my weight was far more *psychological* than physical.

When I did the internal work and came to terms with my childhood demons, I was finally able to get on board the self-care/self-love train and I lost those ten pounds for good. I have been at a healthy weight for over thirty years now and am grateful that I can do almost all the physical activities that I choose to do.

It is my strongest desire to see the same for you!

There are many reasons why people gain more weight than is easy to lose. But starting here, starting today, those reasons don't have to control you. There *is* a systematic way to approach weight loss and there *are* many fitness professionals who specialize in helping people who need to lose 50 pounds or more.

Admittedly, I am not one of them. However, what I have found with my clients is that when an overweight person decides to allow herself/himself to follow their heart and learn the various techniques revealed in this book, it can guide one to take charge of their physical future.

The methods I am presenting here have succeeded time and time again.

Having said all that, the potential physical dangers of being overweight (or "too thick," as my younger daughter said when she put on 30 unwanted pounds one year) are too many and too serious to be ignored:

- Heart Disease
- Type 2 Diabetes
- High Blood Pressure
- Joint Pain
- Stroke
- Sleep Apnea
- Shortness of Breath
- Osteoarthritis
- Gall Bladder Disease or Gallstones
- Some Cancers
- Irritable Bowel Syndrome
- Leaky Gut
- Kidney Disease
- Clinical Depression and/or Anxiety
- Pain from Movement
- Lethargy

Having just one of these disorders interferes with how life is supposed to be lived. Having two or three, which is more typical for those in the "thick" category, takes away any semblance of control or freedom of choice in conducting your life.

When the health of your body dictates the choices you make for your life, it is time to reclaim your independence and free will. Recognizing your right to be healthy for as long as you wish is a decision only you can make, but once you decide, then all you have to do is choose a technique and follow the steps. **It's the *decision to change* that is the toughest step. The implementation of the decision is simply following the rules of the game.**

Before making your decision, there are quite a few things to think about and insights to understand about food in general. And, of course, there is the emotional element that must come first. The most critical part of your food relationship is determining why you eat the way you do. If you have struggled with obesity for some time, the most critical piece to losing the weight forever is to understand why you overate in the first place. I have seen far too many cases of gastric bypass surgery patients losing hundreds of pounds only to gain much of the weight back, since the emotional reason for the obesity was never resolved. The inner demons need to be put to rest before venturing onto a healthier way to be for life.

In this book I offer ideas, plans and suggestions for you to consider. I think the hardest part for most is knowing which path to choose! When something grabs hold of you – when you feel an emotional response to a certain suggestion or passage – pay close attention! It's a sign that both you and your body have found a personal link to a path that will make it easier for you to implement meaningful changes. And don't be afraid to align yourself with a professional who can work with you to implement these methods for your particular situation. It's a great investment in yourself and your future health!

A QUICK WORD ABOUT BINGE EATING

It has taken some time, but binge eating has finally been identified as a legitimate psychological disorder. (It affects more people than anorexia and bulimia combined, and those two disorders have been treated in the psychological community for decades.) Ironically, those who are obese are not necessarily binge eaters and binge eaters are not necessarily obese.

It affects men and women almost equally, and it's not the same as overeating. Granted, when you are on a binge, you are overeating. But, when you are overeating, you are not necessarily on a binge.

Binge eating disorder more often develops in middle age or retirement, when it is increasingly more difficult to lose weight.

Binge eating involves the eater's inability to stop eating. Oftentimes, the eater will set out a specific grouping of food and then just start to eat. In many cases, they will not finish the binge until all the food is gone, regardless of how full they are.

The reason for binge eating has nothing to do with food. Food is simply the vehicle that is used in the mindset's search for appeasement. Reasons for a binge are often because the eater is trying to avoid feeling a certain emotion. By eating, the temporary fix of the yumminess of the food helps to dispel the negative emotions they are, in fact, trying to avoid. Once the binge is over and the food is gone, they are still faced with the emotions they were trying to avoid, but now they also have the guilt and shame from the binge. Never mind the overwhelming discomfort from eating too much! And the cycle goes on.

I, personally, have dabbled in binge eating. I say dabbled as it never really grabbed ahold of me as a vehicle for suppressing my emotions. But there certainly were times when I wanted to bury my feelings, got myself a half-gallon of ice cream (French vanilla) and ate it all in one sitting. I let go of this tool after my first child when I had gained 65 pounds in the pregnancy – *lots* of ice cream was consumed!

The good news is that now there are psychologists and therapists trained in helping people with "Binge Eating Disorder" and most health insurance companies recognize it as a mental health issue. There is help out there with people who understand, so if I am speaking to you, please help yourself. It is not a sustainable way of life as it will take over your health and you will lose control of your physicality, which you do not want to do.

In the meantime, should you find yourself down that path and about to over-indulge, or you are in the middle of a binge and a brief glimpse of sanity crosses your mind, STOP what you are doing. Sit back. Close your eyes. Take a deep breath, very slowly – inhaling through your nose and exhaling through your mouth. Do it again. Repeat a few more times. Now, open your eyes. Do you really want to continue doing what you are doing? If so, then dive in. If the pause has helped you to stop this one, pack it all up and throw it in the trash. Give yourself a big hug of self-love for choosing you!

Remember, the most influential way you can *Thrive to 95* is to take control of your behavior. And eating this way is just not supportive of that mission.

So, now that the help is available, do everything you can to get the help you need to put binge eating behind you.

NO MORE DIETS – WELCOME TO A LIFESTYLE!

It was my older daughter's idea. "Mom, I want to be vegan."

She was in college and when she made this declaration, I agreed it was a healthy direction to take. Upon reflection, I'm not sure what I was thinking regarding the control of choices and behaviors of a 21-year-old living the single life in New York City. More importantly, at the time, I had no idea the discipline it takes to be vegan. But, in the supportive role that I play in her life, I said, "Great! I'll do it too!" It was the summer after her junior year in college, and we both went vegan.

Eleven years later, I will say it is the best "diet" I have ever been on. I have shared my weight journey, so you know I have tried a plethora of "diets." Many work for a while, but when you return to "normal" eating, statistics say 95% of us gain the weight back. This is not something new and I am sure you have either been down this road or know others who have. That is what you hear – the diet did work, but I gained the weight back as soon as I stopped it. That was my story too – for many years.

Veganism is my lifestyle choice because it is what works best for me. Admittedly, it is not easy, but the rewards are many. Being vegan means I do not eat any animals, fish or products from animals, such as dairy products or eggs. By giving up these food groups, I need to get my protein from other sources such as beans, legumes, nuts, seeds, soy, a multitude of vegetables and other protein-heavy foods. And by limiting my diet to these foods, it was much easier to pass up the desserts and snacks I loved. Although many sweet foods and simple carb foods are vegan, the vegan guidelines provided me with the discipline I needed to cut back or eliminate those sugar sources and succeed.

Veganism is what works for me. It has helped me stay healthy and maintain conscience eating for years. It's not for everybody. What program will work for you? What guidelines will support your lifestyle?

HOW TO BEGIN YOUR FOOD CHOICE JOURNEY

Before embarking on changing the way you eat or approach food, there is some basic information you should consider. These warnings are based on what is best for your health. If you choose to adopt these guidelines on a regular basis, you will know that you are doing what is best for your body.

GENETICALLY ENGINEERED/MODIFIED FOOD – GMOS (Bioengineered Food)[37]

There is a lot of rumbling out there about Genetically Modified Organisms – GMOs. The farmers, government and chemical companies are defensive, saying that there is nothing wrong with them. There are others that say there is a whole lot wrong with them.

GMOs are foods which are created to achieve a desired trait, such as resistance to insects or pesticides, but little research has been done to determine the potential health risks. "As genetically modified (GM) foods are starting to intrude in our diet, concerns have been expressed regarding GM food safety. Animal toxicity studies with certain GM foods have shown that they may toxically affect several organs and systems. The review of these studies should not be conducted separately for each GM food, but, according to the effects exerted on certain organs, it may help us create a better picture of the possible health effects on human beings. The results of most studies with GM foods indicate that they may cause some common toxic effects such as hepatic, pancreatic, renal, or reproductive effects and may alter the hematological, biochemical, and immunologic

---

[37] As of January 1, 2022, the term GMO, genetically modified organism, has been relabeled as bioengineered food. As this is newer vocabulary for the same thing, I am maintaining the GMO term throughout this book so as not to confuse the reader.

parameters. However, many years of research with animals and clinical trials are required for this assessment."[38]

My belief is that in order to be the best healthy you, you *must have a strong immune system*. In order to have a strong immune system, you must eat healthfully. In order to eat healthfully, you need to be aware of what you are up against in the food industry so that you can make the best choices for your body. I am passionate about the poisoning of our food supply and GMOs are just a small part of it. Keep in mind, most of the studies being done since the above statement was made are to the nutritional quality and the direct damage of GMO foods to the body. They do not address the chemical pesticides that are sprayed on the GMO crops, but simply the integrity of the GMO food itself.

Again, we turn to the history of Monsanto and the introduction of the weed killer Roundup. Monsanto, which created Agent Orange (an herbicide used in the Vietnam War to kill the overgrowth of plant life in the jungles where the fighting was taking place) created a milder herbicide after the war: glyphosate. Glyphosate kills weeds, so farmers spray it generously around their crops. In addition, Monsanto has genetically engineered many foods so they will NOT die from the glyphosate. So genetically modified foods, sprayed with Roundup weed poison, are in your grocery stores and, most likely, being ingested by you and your family.

The current list of GMO foods from the US Department of Agriculture includes: corn products, including high fructose corn syrup (an additive in many foods), soy (tofu and tempeh, as well as other foods found in many ingredient lists), sugar beets, papaya, zucchini, potatoes, alfalfa, eggplant, summer squash, pineapple, salmon, rapeseed (from which canola oil is derived) and apples. Keep in mind that cattle and poultry eat soy and corn products as well, so unless you are eating organic meat, you are ingesting GMO byproducts via the animal consumed. The safest way to eat any of these and other foods is to buy organic. At least for now, no organic fruits or vegetables are sprayed with Roundup, or glyphosate.

---

[38] nih.org (National Institutes of Health), National Library of Medicine, "Health Risks of Genetically Modified Foods," 2009

Surprisingly, there has not been a GMO created for wheat. However, there is still a huge market for Monsanto in the wheat growing business. Fields are sprayed with glyphosate before planting to make sure there are no weeds in the soil. Then, in order to expedite the harvesting process, fields are sprayed to dry and kill the crop more quickly so that the plants can be harvested two weeks sooner. Which means that the whole wheat bread sold in the store, while not genetically modified, has been sprayed with glyphosate unless it is labeled organic. ("Whole wheat" is a misleading term, by the way. Whole wheat is not a whole grain because it gets processed to make the flour to make the bread. There is nothing whole about the grain used.)

Because of the heavily-funded lobbying efforts of Monsanto and the other chemical companies involved in these toxic practices, there is no labeling for us to know which foods are, in fact, genetically modified. This is why reading your labels is so important, to make sure that none of these foods is part of the ingredients included in the non-organic food you are buying.

According to the US Department of Agriculture, 85%-90% of all US soybeans, sugar beets and corn crops are genetically modified by Monsanto and other GMO producers. How on earth did Monsanto get so much power to control so much of our food supply?

A letter from The Hague dated October 18, 2016, reprinted by the Organic Consumers Association, states: "We are today in the midst of a battleground for two very different approaches to agriculture. One is the agro-ecological approach based on the use of open source traditional seeds based on biodiversity and living in harmony with nature. The other is the mechanistic world of an industrial system based on monocultures, one-way extraction and the use of pesticides, poisons and GMOs where chemical cartels compete to take over our agriculture and food systems, destroying our ecosystems along the way."[39]

---

[39] *Brochure for the People's Assembly,* The Hague, "Seeds of Freedom – Navdanya," October 14, 2016

The bottom line is that GMOs and glyphosate are all potentially wreaking havoc on your immune system. Due to the lack of testing on the toxic effect that genetically-mutated food could have on the food itself, the potential for new toxins being released in the human body upon consumption is unknown, but this potential is feared to exist by FDA scientists. Due to the genetic exchange of one food with another and no regulated GMO labeling on the food to show that it exists, there is risk of someone with an allergy to one food consuming a GMO food and having a severe reaction to it due to the genetic mutation with the allergy-causing food. There is also a risk of resistance to antibiotics. Because most GMO foods contain "antibiotic resistance markers," too much consumption may severely weaken our immune system. Other studies have shown increased risk of colon, breast and prostate cancers.[40]

According to the Institute for Responsible Technology, doctors who put patients on a non-GMO diet found patients quickly getting better with "dramatic results from a variety of different diseases and disorders" - digestive disorders being the most notable, but also brain fog, fatigue, weight and many more. Over 3,200 subscribers who responded to a survey from the Institute for Responsible Technology described an improvement in 28 conditions after stopping GMO food ingestion.[41]

For more in-depth information about GMOs, please visit the websites or Facebook Groups of The Non-GMO Project, The Center for Food Safety, March Against Monsanto, The Environmental Working Group, Institute for Responsible Technology and The Food Revolution.

---

[40] centerforfoodsafety.org, "GE Food and Your Health"
[41] responsibletechnology.org/gmo-dangers/, "GMOs and Roundup are Dangerous" (video)

> ### OPEN SESAME – THE STORY OF SEEDS
>
> When this documentary film was made in 2014, 82% of the seeds throughout the world were owned by corporations, not farmers. Organic farmers are losing the rights to plant their own seeds because companies like Monsanto, a chemical company, are controlling all the rights to the seeds of certain foods.
>
> Also, according to the Food and Agriculture Organization, approximately 90% of crop varieties grown just 100+ years ago are now extinct. In 1901, there were 288 varieties of beets – now there are 17. There were 497 varieties of lettuce and now there are 36. Sweet corn had 307 varieties and today 12. And as for wheat, there were thousands of varieties and most are near extinction now.
>
> The USDA estimates that 94% of soy and 88% of corn in the United States is genetically modified – that means controlled by Monsanto and the GMO producers. Since 1970, 20,000 seed companies have been bought up, leaving the seed business in the United States hanging on for dear life. Without control of the seeds, there can be no control of future produce.

ORGANIC VS. CONVENTIONAL FOODS

The easiest way to avoid GMOs is to always eat organic. Not just fruits and vegetables, but meat and dairy also. The most common reasons for NOT eating organic are availability and affordability.

AVAILABILITY

I am very spoiled in my corner of the United States. Every week in the summer and winter I get local organic produce within 10 miles from my home. I understand most of you are not that fortunate. Availability is a problem, but I do believe that many areas have farmers' markets. First check to see if that farmer's market is, in fact, organic. Because getting certified as organic is extremely expensive. Many farms may be organic, but not certified. Or, they may have a combination of organic and conventional offerings. Just ask. If you visit them in the summer months, ask the farmers what they do in the winter in terms of organic production and offerings. Spread out from your normal go-to farmers' market and see if there are others just a little bit further away that provide year-round greenhouse farming. Even though I have an organic farm ¼ mile from my home, I found my year-round farmer in the next town.

If that fails, check out your chain grocery stores. My local chain store, which is one of over 400 stores throughout New England, New York and New Jersey, offers its own organic brand. And because the food is their brand, it is less expensive. Give your local chain store a chance and if they are not offering any organic food, maybe you can be the catalyst and ask them to bring organic in.

If availability of organic is still a problem, I urge you to go to the website for the Environmental Working Group, www.ewg.org. The Environmental Working Group offers a couple of lists every year: the "Dirty Dozen" and the "Clean 15." The Dirty Dozen is a list of the most heavily pesticide-sprayed fruits and vegetables. It is highly recommended that those foods should only be eaten if organic. The Clean 15 are those foods that are the least sprayed and, if cannot be found organically, are safer to eat than others not on the list.

AFFORDABILITY

Cost is another factor in eating organic. Believe me; I know the pinch of the pocketbook very well. There was a time when as a single parent I had to rely on food stamps. I would shop in three different grocery stores each week to follow the sales and cut out the individual store coupons just so I could feed my family of four – but we still ate organically.

The real issue is that the price you pay for organic food NOW is a drop in the bucket compared to the cost of poor health down the line. The healthier your immune system from eating organic foods, the less likely you are to develop illness down the road. I can assure you, eating organic will help minimize your medical costs as you get older.

When you eat conventional produce that has been sprayed with herbicides, pesticides and insecticides, both as they are grown and as they are protected in shipping, your body is in a constant battle fighting off all the dangers that those poisons bring to it. Your immune system is constantly working in overdrive to take care of those gremlins and to put your systems back into a balanced state. Unfortunately, that doesn't leave much strength to fight off germs during times like cold and flu seasons. Colds and flu are the most common illnesses that prey on weaker immune systems. And for long term gestation of these toxins, illnesses like cancer, multiple sclerosis and Parkinson's disease can manifest.

When you eat organic, you are giving your body permission to focus on the healthy nutrients, empowering your immune system to keep you healthy and strong. It certainly works for me! Aside from having Covid before everyone else did, I bet it has been ten or more years since I have had a cold and I don't even remember the last time I had the flu or bronchitis, or been bed-ridden in general. I just don't get sick. I attribute that to my strong immune system which has been built up over the years. My bout with Covid lasted a mere five days, but it was brutal.

It is worth noting that much of the scientific data comparing conventional and organic foods focus on nutrition content. The data report on produce shows that both conventional and organic produce are equal in nutrient density. Apples to apples and squash to squash, so to speak. There is some ongoing research to determine if either is *more* nutritious, but there is no conclusive evidence to date. In other words, the poisons do not seem to affect the nutrition content of the produce, but they certainly have an effect on the overall health of the consumer.

There are quite a few regulations that must be met in order for foods to be labeled organic. This is true for all organics, be it produce, meat or dairy.

We have learned about produce, but paying attention to meat and dairy is equally important. According to the Mayo Clinic, organic farming practices for livestock include:

- Healthy living conditions and access to the outdoors
- Pasture feeding for at least 30 percent of livestock's nutritional needs during grazing season
- Organic foods for animals
- Vaccinations

If and when you choose to eat non-free range, non-organic beef, you need to understand what cows are fed. Remember, if they are eating it, so are you!

According to the Organic Consumers Association[42], cows are legally fed:

- Same species meat remnants, including hair, skin, hooves and blood
- Remains of other potentially diseased animals
- Manure and other animal waste
- Plastic pellets to help digestion and replace the lack of fiber in their diet
- Corn and other grains their systems were not designed to digest
- Massive amounts of antibiotics to offset the diseases they may ingest from other animals, or diseases that are created by their own bodies in an effort to process the undigestible food they are fed

Again, I urge you to find local meat and dairy, if at all possible. Asserting that animals have "access to the outdoors" does not necessarily mean Bessie the Cow is walking around in a field, grazing to her heart's content. That scenario is more likely if Bessie is local. Organic is always better in these categories because the animals are being fed organic food that will then pass on to you. But you do want free range, too, so that you are eating cows that have not been confined to a stall so small they cannot turn around and have had a more stress-free life.

---

[42] organicconsumersassociation.org/News, "They Eat What? What Are They Feeding Animals on Factory Farms?"

The bottom line is that organic food is simply healthier than non-organic.

When you can control what goes on your plate, organic food should be your choice.

THE HAVES AND THE HAVE-NOTS

There are hundreds, if not thousands, of books telling you what to eat and what not to eat. While it is nice to see the tide turning, it can be difficult to determine what diet is the best for *you*. Many diets have come and gone, some much better than others. It is important to choose one that cooperates with your body and that provides the most nutrients for the least number of calories. It is important to do your homework when choosing a change in your diet.

I am sure you have noticed that people are better educated and informed today and, if paying attention, are aware that there is a healthy way to eat and an unhealthy way to eat. There are certain foods that should be completely avoided or, at the very least, limited in every person's diet. And there are certain foods that, unless allergic, should be included in everyone's diet.

How do you figure out which foods are actually the best ones for you? And what is the difference between a food allergy, food intolerance and food sensitivity? In a very small nutshell, when the immune system reacts badly to a specific protein in the food and your body indicates that reaction with something as mild as a rash or runny nose, you have a food allergy. The most extreme reaction can lead to anaphylaxis shock and death. Food intolerance arises when there is a problem in the digestion of a specific food consumed and may cause gut-related issues and a plethora of other symptoms. Food sensitivity covers all bases and refers to any food that may cause a physiological reaction in your body. The easiest way to know which foods are best for you is to pay attention to your body's reaction to all foods. If there is a discomfort with a specific food, then test it further.

"The Elimination Diet" is truthfully the best and most affordable method. This diet involves giving up one particular food type, let's say DAIRY, for approximately a month and then slowly re-introducing it back into your diet and watching how your body reacts to it. If you have a physical reaction, such as cramping, diarrhea, lethargy, nausea or constipation, then you know that your body is really not too fond of dairy. It would serve you well to ingest as little as possible, if any at all.

Another option is to have your blood tested. Food sensitivity tests cross your blood with a multitude of common foods. They are relatively inexpensive (when you consider the information they are providing that will help support your future health) and determine which foods your body has trouble processing. The lab which I use can test as many as 176 foods, additives and microbes in your diet, pointing out those that might be problematic.[43] In many cases, you have no idea there is a problem with these foods because your body has learned to accommodate them, but not in a good way.

By finding out what foods affect your body most, you learn what foods are causing inflammation in your system. We now know that inflammation is at the root of most diseases and disorders. From cancer to auto-immune disorders, Parkinson's to Alzheimer's, **most disease starts with persistent inflammation**. It makes sense to learn what foods *your body* does not agree with. Then you can start the elimination process more directly, allowing healing and homeostasis (balance) to return. Your overall health improves as your immune system gets stronger and more vital, no longer working hard to stabilize the inflammation. I offer this because I truly believe *this* is the best way to learn about the impact of the foods you eat. You can then easily change your diet for the better.

---

[43] For more information on how and where to get this test, please visit www.TheAgingCoach.com. You can also be tested for molds, candida, additives, preservatives and food coloring, anti-inflammatory agents and antibiotics as well as many herbs and micro-nutrients. There are many tests now available, but be aware that test results from some laboratories may be inaccurate. There is also a specific way to eat prior to the testing that is important so that the results are as precise as they can be.

Whether you decide to get a food sensitivity test or not, there are some foods that are always bad for you. These foods can cause inflammation, speed up aging and support a multitude of diseases:

- Sugar, including high fructose corn syrup
- Artificial sweeteners
- Vegetable oils, including canola oil
- Excessive alcohol
- Soda, including diet soda
- Bread and processed flour, including corn and "whole wheat"
- Pasta
- Dairy
- Genetically modified foods
- All trans fats, such as fried foods, margarine, pastries, shortening, non-dairy coffee creamer

OUR BODIES ARE THE VICTIMS

Our bodies' organs were not made to digest the kinds of food (including what was sprayed on it or fed to it) that are being presented to our digestive systems. Our bodies are doing the best they can, but unless you are eating a strict diet of locally grown, purely organic whole foods (including meat and dairy), there is probably some stress within your intestinal tract and some inflammation somewhere in your body, which is the precursor to disease. That stress and inflammation are affecting the health and well-being of your immune system, which in turn affect your vitality, energy and quality of life. The nutrients in our food determine the quality of the nutrients throughout our body, which create the base for the regeneration of the cells we grow every day. Poor nutrients = poor cell quality = poor cell function. Healthy nutrients = healthy cell function = healthy body. The quality of the nutrients we ingest determines the quality of the cells that run our bodies, which determines the quality of the life that we live.

I state the following emphatically: **There is not one chemical, poison or additive that has been added to or sprayed onto our food that is**

healthy! Please, do not ignore this fact – it is the most important thing you can acknowledge on your journey to aging the healthiest way you can.

Keep in mind that our bodies are also the victims of not just what we eat, but when we eat and how much. Perhaps you have heard the expression, "Eat breakfast like a king, lunch like a prince and dinner like a pauper." This kind of a schedule would best serve the body as well. As a society, however, we have not been trained to eat this way, but rather the reverse. Rather than go through the multitude of ways to change your eating schedule, I offer you this: Recognize that eating your largest meals earlier in the day will better serve your body and your weight. As for dinner, lighten it up and try to eat earlier. My mom *always* ate at 7:00pm. So, in those last 13 years, I ate dinner then to keep her company. After she passed, I slowly made my way to a 5:30 dinner, which I love. Then there is time (for most of the year) to take a walk after dinner.

Yes, that is early, I admit. And, when I go out with friends, needless to say, I eat later. But, after my walk, I relax with a nice glass of wine and a piece of dark chocolate and I am content. I do not get hungry before bed and I am not ravenous when I wake up. Through trial and error, this is what works for me. I only suggest to you, knowing that lighter meals later are better for you, to adjust your dining schedule and menu if you can.

YOUR MICROBIOME – THE GATEWAY TO GOOD HEALTH

For nutritionists, the term "microbiome" has been discussed for years. For you, however, because it was not really recognized to exist until the late 1990s, this may be the first time you have heard of it. Your microbiome is a system of trillions of cells – microorganisms – that live throughout your body consisting of bacteria, fungi, viruses and protozoa. Though mostly related to your gut, the microbiome is also associated with your nose, mouth, skin, and genital area.

It turns out that about 70% of our immune system is located in our gut. Everything we ingest goes through our digestive system and ends up in our gut. It makes sense that the health of our gut is directly influenced by *what we eat*. Below I quote three doctors who specialize in Gut Flora and Gut Microbiome:

Gut flora and gut microbiome consist of "thousands of species of good bacteria [which are] directly connected with your biology all the time, controlling levels of inflammation, the permeability of your intestines or leaky gut … your brain chemistry, your hormones, your metabolism, your nutrient levels, what you absorb and don't absorb."[44]

"I think we will find that the microbiome is important in just about all the chronic diseases that have risen dramatically since World War II, since the widespread use of antibiotics."[45]

"There are huge advances in research where they are finding how the gut microbiome impacts all disease."[46]

And, from the Center of Ecogenetics, "auto-immune diseases such as diabetes, rheumatoid arthritis, muscular dystrophy, multiple sclerosis and fibromyalgia are associated with dysfunction in the microbiome.… Auto-immune diseases appear to be passed in families not by DNA inheritance but by inheriting the family's microbiome."[47]

The microbiome is the combination of all the microorganisms we have in our bodies. Bacteria and viruses are the most easily recognized, but it really consists of ALL the microscopic creatures that live on and in our bodies. There are more than 100 trillion of them. What has been discovered is that the health of these trillions of cells of bacteria in our bodies determines whether we are diseased or not. And the health of these trillions of cells is

---

[44] *Interconnected Series*, Cleveland Clinic for Functional Medicine, Dr. Mark Hyman
[45] Dr. Martin Blaser, Director Microbiome Program, New York University
[46] Datis Kharrazian, PhD, DHSc, Research Fellow, Harvard Medical School
[47] The Center for Ecogenetics and Environmental Health, University of Washington, "Fast Facts About the Human Microbiome," Jan 2014

largely determined by what we have put in our mouths over the decades of our lives.

It is also known that a meal that includes saturated fats and/or a high sugar content imposes on the normal function of the immune system and can enhance inflammation, especially within the few hours following the ingestion.

Science has already proven the negative impact certain foods have on our bodies through studies on asthma and allergies. As we have discussed, cardiovascular disease is said to be mainly preventable. According to recent studies, cancer is more and more often being tied to diet, stress and trauma. Even Alzheimer's and dementia are being linked to what we eat and how we handle our stress.

Many diseases fall under the umbrella of autoimmune disorders. These aren't actually new diseases; they are just considerably more common now.

The latest science is showing the relationship between our diet and these diseases. The foods we are eating have compromised our immune systems so severely that we have built up no defenses, or very weak ones, to fend off these disorders. The only way for our immune system to get strong is to eat the right foods for our body.

Another very important thing to be aware of is the role of antibiotics.

Taking antibiotics plays a huge part in the sickness of our gut and, consequently, our immune system. Antibiotics have a job to do – they kill bacteria when we are sick. Unfortunately, antibiotics kill *all* the kinds of bacteria in our body, the good and the bad, which severely compromises our microbiome and its ability to keep us healthy. (Remember 70%+ of our immune system is in our microbiome.) It can take months, some say a year, to restore our microbiome from just one round of antibiotics. A direct correlation has been drawn between childhood illnesses and antibiotics. Kids are much sicker and have far more allergies now than they did 40 years ago, and the amount of antibiotics prescribed is far greater than ever before. At least 28 percent of antibiotics prescribed in the United States are unnecessary.[48]

Six in 10 adults have a chronic disease and 4 out of every 10 adults have two or more.[49] "By 2025, chronic diseases will affect an estimated 164 million Americans – nearly half of the (estimated) population."[50]

It All Has to Do with Our Gut

What is needed for each and every one of us is an individualistic approach to our gut health. Every single person is unique in the development of their individual microbiome. Because we have grown up with distinct foods and dietary habits, our microbiome is unique to us. What foods are good for me are not necessarily good for you. And true in the reverse: The foods that are bad for me are not necessarily bad for you. It would not matter if we both ate the same diet every day. The foods will affect our systems differently because our systems are unique to us, created from our history of food intake and our environment.

ACID VS. ALKALINE – A BALANCING ACT

Another path to a healthier microbiome and stronger immune system is to eat more foods that are alkaline in nature versus acidic. Acidity promotes inflammation while alkalinity helps to cool things down and keeps the body balanced, forever seeking homeostasis. Again, each of our digestive systems is unique. Some highly acidic foods might not seem to affect you at all, yet the same foods will leave your spouse suffering from heartburn, for instance. Whether you suffer now or not, it's important to recognize the more acid-producing foods and eliminate them from your diet.

Google defines homeostasis as "the tendency toward a relatively stable equilibrium between interdependent elements, especially as maintained

---

[48] cdc.gov (Centers for Disease Control), "Antibiotic Prescribing and Use"
[49] rand.org, *Rand Review,* "Chronic Conditions in America: Price and Prevalence"
[50] fightchronicdisease.org, "The Growing Crisis of Chronic Disease in the U.S."

by physiological processes." Think 8th grade science. Your body is always trying to reach a state of balance. When things are out of balance, you can be darn sure that your body is doing everything it can to stabilize. A visual to help with this is to picture a duck gliding across a pond. Above the water, the duck looks calm and seems to be cruising pretty easily, while below the water we know he is paddling his feet like crazy.

Usually, we do not even feel the stabilization process going on, unless our bodies are really off-kilter. As with most body systems, it is a non-stop, never-ending process.

We can make things a lot easier by eating foods that support homeostasis and are not toxic to our systems. The ability to identify acidic versus alkaline foods is an important tool in your toolbox of healthy-eating tricks.

The fewer acidic foods you eat, the more alkaline your system will be, and therefore the more in balance you are and the closer you are to achieving a state of homeostasis. The closer you get to maintaining homeostasis, the less susceptible you are to disease and illness. Having a neutrally alkaline body allows your body to function at its highest levels. BEGONE fatigue, muscle soreness, digestive issues, heart arrhythmias, headaches, insomnia…and all the other things we address in health today. I am sure you can add to that list!

So, which foods are acidic and which are alkaline? Some you might think are acidic are not. In fact, citrus fruits are alkaline-generating once they've been digested and absorbed. Acid-forming foods include meat, fish, dairy, sugar, coffee, alcohol and most grains.

You might be asking right about now, "Is there *anything* left to eat?!"

Of course there is! Most vegetables and many fruits are alkaline. Cucumbers, watermelon, avocado, spinach, kale, bananas, broccoli and celery are especially alkaline-rich.

No one expects you to eliminate all acidic foods from your diet. The important key here is, if you are going to eat foods in the acidic category, make sure that you are offsetting their level of consumption with vegetables and other alkaline foods.

I recommend you check your alkaline levels. It is easy to do. You can pick up a kit at any local drugstore or order one online. These kits are pH balance test strips designed to analyze your urine and measure your pH balance, or alkaline levels. The ideal level is 7.35 – this falls in the mid-section on the pH scale of 1 to 14.

There are many lists of acid versus alkaline foods out there and not all of them are accurate. Do your research. One site I like is www.liveenergized.com.

A BRIEF HORMONE/DIET CONNECTION

When we are consistently eating an acidic diet and our body is constantly fighting to maintain a state of homeostasis, our systems often have a higher dose of cortisol than needed. Cortisol is the hormone that is produced by our adrenal glands when we are stressed. It is left over from our cave man days of *fight or flight*. Too much cortisol helps the body maintain inflammation and hold onto fat. We have already learned how inflammation is the precursor to many diseases. When higher than normal levels of cortisol are produced on a regular basis, it also wears out your adrenal glands and can cause overall fatigue, often unable to be relieved. High levels of cortisol are simply not good for our bodies or our health.

Additionally, chronic imbalance caused by higher levels of cortisol seems to disrupt the action of two other very critical hormones: leptin and ghrelin.

Leptin is produced by your fat cells and tells your brain when your stomach is full and no longer needs to eat. You are satiated.

Ghrelin is the hormone, released by several sources, that tells you when you are hungry.

Needless to say, if these two hormones fail to accurately tell your brain how you feel, it leads to either over-eating or depriving yourself of food when fuel is needed. Neither one of these is a good thing.

Our endocrine system is a critical piece in keeping all our systems in balance. It allows the hormones to maintain balance and facilitates the conversations that take place throughout the body. When imbalance occurs and the endocrine system is working overtime, our body has no choice but to reach exhaustion. Controlling stress is one way to help keep hormone levels in check.

IN CONCLUSION...

"You are what you eat" might be something you have heard throughout your life.

If you have, it is my hope you recognize how true that statement is. If this is a new concept to you, I really hope you have benefitted from the information shared here. I personally believe "You are what you eat" is the single most important lesson we can learn in regard to our health. Our food consumption, from childhood to aging adulthood, is in such a bad state that I am on a mission to educate and wake everyone up to this reality.

In a world of air pollution, contaminated water supplies, the proliferation of pesticides on our crops and poison being fed to the animals we eat, **we need to pay a lot more attention to what we put into our bodies!**

If you truly want to Thrive to 95, it is critical that you allow your body to operate at peak efficiency. This can ONLY be done if it is fed the foods that support that efficiency. It is also very possible that once you have a steady healthy diet and your body responds in a positive way to the changes you have made, that you may be able to reduce any medication that you are on. You certainly will offset the potential for future medication recommendations!

I am fully aware that it is not easy to make the changes suggested. Putting too much pressure on yourself only leads to frustration and then to failure and more stress. Taking baby steps is the best way to succeed - take your time, but start *somewhere* in making these transitions. Slow, steady, positive change keeps you heading in the right direction. A marathon runner does not start out running the marathon – pace yourself and keep moving forward. Your body's sole purpose is to provide you with the healthiest vessel it can to let you live your life to its fullest. It is your mind's responsibility to support the body in every way it can.

CHAPTER 9 RECAP

1) For thousands of years, mankind was doing just fine with the quality of available food. In the 1950s, to help accommodate a growing population, supermarkets cropped up and bulk food production was the new wave of providing food to the masses.
2) Around the same time, convenience became important, which supported the production of processed foods.
3) To accommodate the increase in food production, the government helped subsidize the farmers to grow more and more food.
4) To facilitate the increase in food production, pesticides, herbicides and insecticides were introduced into the foods.
5) In 1974, post-Vietnam, the manufacturer of Agent Orange, Monsanto, created a milder version to be sprayed on these huge fields of crops to allay weed growth.
6) The long term effects of these toxins were never really studied; however, we are now seeing the effects in the poor health of most Americans.
7) Most processed foods have little to no nutritional value and are mostly understood to be treated by the body as if they are sugar.
8) It is very important to read your food labels, not just for ingredients, but for sugar content. The carbohydrates, minus dietary fiber, in any processed food should be counted as sugar.
9) Sugar ingestion produces the feel-good hormones of serotonin and dopamine which help to create sugar addiction.
10) The determination that cholesterol was bad for us in the 1970s led to the food industry stripping bad fats out of the food which took the

flavor with it. To enhance the taste in many foods, sugar was added and the obesity epidemic began.

11) Whether you have ten pounds or one hundred pounds to lose, your success will only come when you realize why you overeat in the first place.

12) Binge eating is now recognized as a mental health disorder and if you suffer from this disorder, you can get help more easily these days. Binge eating has nothing to do with the food, but learning the reason for the practice will help you to overcome it.

13) There are no studies of the long-term effects of bioengineered foods (GMOs), but the research to date suggests the havoc that they are wreaking on our bodies.

14) Because of mass production, the variety of crops/seeds available today has decreased dramatically from 100 years ago. Ninety percent of the crop varieties grown then are now extinct.

15) Though the difference in nutrient content may be negligible, the difference between the effects of organic vs. conventional crops on your health due to pesticides is dramatic.

16) Though buying organic can be more expensive, it is a fraction of the price you could pay in medical costs from decades of conventional food consumption.

17) Most disease begins from persistent inflammation. Persistent inflammation is supported by an unhealthy gut, which is created by the food you eat over time and your body's reaction to the food you are eating.

18) Your body can react negatively to food through an allergy, food intolerance or food sensitivity. Taking a food sensitivity test is an excellent way to determine how your body reacts to certain foods.

19) Antibiotics kill both good and bad bacteria and it can take up to a year for the microbiome to recuperate from one dose of antibiotics. At least 70% of your immune system is located in the gut, so that dose of antibiotics has weakened your immune system for months.

20) Balance your diet with alkaline foods to offset the typically higher intake of acidic foods.

21) It is critical to pay a lot more attention to what you put into your mouth if you truly want to *Thrive to 95!*

Chapter 10
THE MIND-BODY PARTNERSHIP

"Life is what you make it. Always has been. Always will be."

Grandma Moses

I was standing in front of my house, close to the road, weeding out the tiger lilies.

Bend over. Lean on one knee. Pull and pull. Lean on other knee. Pull and pull. Repeat.

I asked myself, "What would be the most beneficial position for my body that will allow me to get this job done efficiently?"

The answer I heard was, "Get your butt on the ground!" So, I did. I made sure I was in a clear enough spot within the lilies and I sat down.

Reach and pull. Reach and pull.

There was *no* stress of movement anywhere in my body!

This exchange was a result of paying attention and asking my body what it wanted. I could sense that I was putting an unnecessary strain on my back, so I asked my body what I could do to fix it. I got my answer. The lilies got weeded efficiently and my back was delighted! Now I could move on to my next chore.

Typically, we go through our day doing all our tasks with no consideration at all about the toll it takes on our bodies. But if we hurt ourselves or overdo it, the body talks back to us in the form of aches and pains. *Then* we pay attention. I would like to propose doing this communication in reverse. When you have a task at hand that will put exertion on the body, take a minute to pause and think how it can be done with utmost consideration to the physicality of both the task and the body's involvement.

There really is a partnership between you and your body. You need your body to be as strong and flexible as possible for it to perform all the necessary activities that you do throughout the day. You think of something to do and your body responds.

You expect your body to respond.

Your body performs a multitude of other tasks throughout each day that we don't even think about. These are so automatic, we just simply do them.

YOUR BODY IS A WONDERLAND: THE BODY'S SYSTEMS AND HOW THEY WORK[51]

Without going into great detail, I want to outline the systems of the body so that you can better understand or be reminded of the plethora of functions that the body does for you, most of which you can't feel and of which you are unaware. It is important to understand what the body does for us to help gain a better respect for its ever-ready presence and never-ending functionality.

The Circulatory System, or the cardiovascular system. A remarkable interconnected freeway bringing oxygen-rich blood from the lungs to the

---

[51] Cleveland Clinic, Mayo Clinic, PubMed Health – National Library of Medicine, Live Science and the Merck Manuals

heart, then to the rest of the body so that all systems can relish in the oxygen. This happens, on average, 12 – 20 times per minute. The more efficient your circulation, the fewer breaths are needed to accomplish the same enrichment. The oxygen-rich blood also contains nutrients from the food and drink we ingest – the healthier the ingredients, the healthier the blood.

The Digestive System basically consists of the mouth, the throat, the esophagus, the stomach, and the small and large intestines. We chew food in our mouth, swallow and the food passes through our throat down our esophagus into our stomach. The more chewed our food, the easier it is digested. The stomach acids go to work and break down what it has received, then passes it into our small intestines and then to our large intestines (which total about 25 feet in length). The important part to remember is that through digestion, nutrients are extracted from the food and dispersed throughout the body. The quality of the food ingested determines the quality of the nutrients dispersed.

The Endocrine System is composed of a multitude of organs that secrete hormones. These hormones regulate everything from our metabolism to our sexual organs. The endocrine system is an intricate system of glands that communicate and regulate the hormones that need to be secreted, telling them when they need to be secreted and at what levels. The hormones do more than regulate our metabolism, they are what trigger our stress levels, enhance our sexual callings, oversee our digestion, stabilize our blood pressure and heart rate, stimulate our muscle tone – the list goes on and on!

The Excretory System involves the elimination of waste product from the body in the body's effort to maintain homeostasis. The most recognizable functions of homeostasis are sweating, urination, and defecation. Sweating is a form of excretion where the glands in the skin open and water (sweat) is released in an effort to cool the body down when it gets overheated. Sweat can also be released when we are excessively nervous – our emotions trigger the sweat glands. Sweating is an excellent way to detoxify the body from all outside pollutants absorbed through the air we breathe, through the pores in our skin and from the toxins in our food. Urination eliminates excess water from our bodies. It also eliminates waste from digestion and cell degeneration, using the kidneys in the process. Defecation comes from the large intestines, removing solid waste from the foods we eat.

The Immune System. In my opinion, this is the most important system we have supporting our health and wellbeing. It is your internal army of cells whose sole purpose is to protect you from dangerous outside sources that can damage and destroy other systems in your body. A strong immune system can defeat germs and toxins in some, cancer in others. An immune system is only as strong as the cells within it. Strong cells are created through diet, exercise and healthy living – all the things you are learning about in this book.

The Integumentary System has everything to do with our outer layer and protective covering – our skin. Our hair and nails are also included, as well as some glands and nerves. The main function of this system is to help the interaction among the body's other systems to protect and preserve the wellbeing of the body. Our skin acts as a natural wall of protection for all the operations of the body, assists with the regulation of body temperature and helps to protect against disease.

The Lymphatic System works together with the immune system in supporting our good health. It operates through a system of nodes, or pockets of fluid, and travels node-to-node through lymph vessels throughout the body. The lymph fluid transports nutrients, proteins and oxygen that nourish the body's tissues. But along with the good comes the bad, as bacteria and cancer cells can also be transported through the lymphatic system of vessels and sometimes cluster in the nodes. Though a defense system is intact to eliminate this bad aspect, our overall health and strength plays a key role in the success of this defense system.

The Musculoskeletal System. This system is the one most impacted by aging. Muscle tissue tends to atrophy as we age. This impacts our strength and how we carry ourselves, as well as the efficiency of joint flexibility. Bone tissue tends to weaken as we age which contributes to osteoporosis and a greater potential for broken bones. Our spinal tissue shrinks and we get shorter. Our shoulders tend to round more if we don't pay attention to our posture. Ironically, even though it is the most aging impacted system, it is also the one system over which we have the most control.

The Nervous System consists of the autonomic nervous system (involuntary) and the peripheral nervous system (intentional action). Activities such as heartbeat, breathing, metabolism and organ-to-organ communication are all involved in the autonomic system. Movement and external intentional action of our arms and legs, hands and feet are a part of the peripheral system. The efficiency of the entire system is based on the efficacy of each of its parts: clear brain, clear lungs, clean gastro-intestinal tract, flexible joints, strong muscles, etc. All of these are involved in the relative level of performance of your central nervous system.

The Reproductive System consists of the necessary organs in the procreation of the species. Men and women grow through puberty into adulthood within their second decade of life. Sexuality and the level of involvement or use of the reproductive system's organs vary from man to man and woman to woman. The joining of the sperm from a man and the egg from a woman, beginning as a microscopic dot and nine months later becoming a human being, is extraordinary and one of the most awesome abilities we humans have.

The Respiratory System is the exchange of gases in which we take in oxygen and send it to all parts of the body, and then remove the waste gas carbon dioxide. Our respiratory system must be functioning at its peak at all times, or we can die. In only a three-to-five minute period of no oxygen exchange, our brains can be incapacitated forever. The intricacy of the process – oxygen entering the lungs, going through the lung capillaries into the blood, being transported to the heart and throughout the body in cooperation with the circulatory system, and carbon dioxide being collected and transported to the lungs for exhalation – is miraculous. This exchange happens up to twenty times per minute.

I truly hope that you took the time to read through this summary of just some of the interactions with which your body functions every minute of every day. It is important to recognize the elaborate, interconnecting set of activities that is going on throughout your body continuously. You are not even aware of most of these processes as they are occurring. Consider that these are your body's responsibilities and it is living up to its end of the bargain to keep you functioning every moment you are alive.

And, on top of all these subconscious functions, we also want our bodies to climb stairs, weed the garden, clean the house, do the laundry, wash the dishes, sit, stand, drive a car, and stand and sit some more! Just imagine how many tasks you demand of your body each day!! We expect it to do everything we ask. More often than not, it does!

WHAT IS YOUR ROLE IN ALL OF THIS?

What we think about pretty much runs the show. I am sure you have heard the quotes, "What you think, you become" (attributed to Buddha), and "You become what you think about" (attributed to Earl Nightingale). I have a favorite version attributed to Henry Ford, "If you think you can or you think you can't, you're right!"

Our brain is in charge of all that we think and do. Our brain is also in charge of how we move our bodies and what we feed our bodies. Our body has no power over the mind. It is astonishing to think of all the systems that operate subconsciously throughout the body, without which we would die. And yet for all our conscious behavior involving the body, the body has no control. Our conscious mind is in charge of the doing, and the doing requires your body.

So, how can you make sure that your body will be capable of what you ask? Let me ask that another way: What is your role in this mind-body partnership and how can you play your part in the best possible way? After all, we are talking about your life partner here. There is not another human on the planet with whom you will spend more time than yourself. Doesn't it make sense to develop a way to better understand how your body is speaking and what your body is telling you? Your body knows what it needs, but are you listening? There is a communication going on, but do you understand it? Are you paying attention? Are you an active participant in it?

I offer you a very simple way to hear what your body is telling you: Ask *why*.

When a sensation happens in your body, ask what just happened to make you feel it. For example, you eat pizza and get heartburn afterwards. Your body is trying to tell you that this kind of food does not agree with your digestive system and that you should not be eating it. Instead of hearing this message, the typical response is to take an antacid tablet to calm your stomach down and stop the heartburn. Your body is saying eating pizza is not good for your body. It's saying, "Please don't eat any more pizza. My digestive system can't take it. That's why I am giving you heartburn. Please, don't eat any more pizza." But do you listen?

By itself, getting heartburn after eating pizza is not going to kill you. However, the acidic reaction from your body, compounded with other damage from other foods and behaviors you do over time, certainly can.

Research published in a 2017 Journal of the American Medical Association addressed this very topic. A study from 2012 of 702,308 cardio-related deaths revealed that approximately 45% of those deaths were *directly related* to the foods that the individuals did or did not eat.[52]

Your body is communicating with you for your better health. How else can the body tell you to stop eating foods that are difficult for it to process? Its only choice is a physical reaction. What you THINK about that physical reaction is up to you, not your body. Whether you choose not to eat the offending food again or take an antacid is up to you, not your body.

Here is another communication from the body that is very often misunderstood. Constipation. Constipation is usually the body's way of

---

[52] jamanetwork.com (Journal of the American Medical Association), "Association Between Dietary Factors and Mortality from Heart Disease, Stroke, and Type 2 Diabetes in the United States," March 7, 2017

telling you that it needs more fluids and fiber. I honestly was not aware of this, and have discovered that so many others aren't either! I spent most of my adult life constipated (now there's something to openly admit to the world!) I went to a number of doctors and was always trying different kinds of laxatives to keep my system functioning. Through my journey learning how to have the healthiest lifestyle, I discovered a very simple solution: drink more water and eat the right foods! For me, personally, that meant saying goodbye to meat and dairy. Constipation is a thing of the past for me - forever. Had I understood the communication from my body in the first place, the problem could have been easily solved in my teens versus in my fifties! As an aside, not one of those doctors ever mentioned drinking more water or changing my diet!

The mind is responsible for translating the body's communication. We often recruit a professional to help us identify what is wrong and what we can do about it. Regardless of the recommendation of the professional, your mind is still the part of you that will react and take action. You can accept what the professional says, you can get another opinion, you can try alternative medical advice, or you can do your own research and be your own best advocate. Whatever forward motion you decide to take, it is always a result of the mind taking charge of what happens to the body.

AND THEN THERE'S MENOPAUSE...

If you are to live past the age of 55 or so, you will go through menopause. There are actually 4 stages to menopause. There is pre-menopause – the time before any symptoms begin. Before you know it, you are perimenopausal – when your periods are definitely erratic and less frequent, and menopausal symptoms begin to appear: cramping, hot flashes, headaches, mood swings, face flushing, fatigue, bloating, weight gain, night sweats, insomnia, lack of libido and more. Your body is definitely telling you that things are changing. Then, of course, there is menopause, when your periods have stopped for more than 12 months and they are never coming back. The final stage is post-menopause when the ovaries are done for good and the hormone changes can become evident.

I was very fortunate when I went through menopause. After a year or so of erratic periods, I had one last period, a 30-second hot flash, and I was done. None of the horrific symptoms I would read about or hear about from friends. Luckily, I was blessed with no expectations. My mom, who had horrible periods throughout her life, ironically breezed right through menopause, so that was my expectation. That it was no big deal. I think that mindset helped me to have no fear or concern.

If you think about it, the ten-year timeframe surrounding menopause is chock full of communications between the mind and the body. Each woman's experience is unique to them and is based on the relationship that they have with their own body. It has everything to do with listening to what the body needs each day, each hour, and sometimes, each minute. Respect the huge changes that are taking place and give your body a fair chance to adjust with each stage. Be patient with yourself and your body. The more you can keep your mind and your body in direct communication and on the same wavelength, the smoother the transitions can be.

The menopause decade is going to happen no matter what. My suggestion is to keep an open mind and a patient heart and listen to your body and what it is trying to say. And maybe you, too, can breeze right through.

WHO'S THE PRETTY GIRL IN THAT MIRROR THERE?

I'm going to let you in on a little secret: How you feel about what you look like is all in your head. Literally! And, it's in *your* head, no one else's. Body image has been controlled by the media and Hollywood since we were born. It's all about what "they" look like and dress like. Unfortunately, "approximately 80% of middle-aged women and 60% of older women are dissatisfied with their body."[53]

At this stage of our lives, let's turn the tables a bit. Let's believe in a positive body image based on how we feel and how we can use our bodies without repercussions. Let's feel good about ourselves because of the kind of person

---

[53] *IDEA Fitness Journal*, Winter 2022

we have become, not because we have gained a few pounds around the middle. Let's focus on creating a healthy body and being proud of how that makes us feel. Rather than focus on what our bodies look like, focus on what our bodies do for us.

Recognize that gravity has a little bit more power now, so our physicality might not be exactly the way we want it. But by taking more control of the choices we make, the power we have and the thoughts we think, the daily effort can help to put our egos aside and focus on the positive thoughts and rewarding tasks we choose to include in our lives.

And because you now realize that you and your body are partners in this life, you know you are not alone. You are there for each other. You are each other's support system. But because you run the show, it's your thoughts that will determine how you feel.

WILL YOU BE A VICTIM OR AN ADVOCATE?

The success of the partnership with your body all depends on the role you choose. The body has no choice in the matter. It will cope with, flourish in, or fall apart based on what you decide.

So, I ask you a very important question now. How much responsibility will you take in your body's caregiving?

Our health care system is set up so that when people get ill or have symptoms of illness and disease, we go to the doctor, get a diagnosis, get a recommendation (often in the form of a prescription), abide by that recommendation and most of the time we "get better"… until the next round of illness. This is the path for the majority of us. I want to step in and be a change-maker here.

Have you ever wondered, "Was there anything I could have done that might have let me avoid this entire scenario and not get sick in the first place?"

THE MIND-BODY PARTNERSHIP

Your immune system is responsible for the maintenance of your good health. Its job is to fight off any foreign germ, virus, bacteria or disease that befalls your body and dispel it from your physicality. Depending on the virility of your immune system, you either get sick, you do not get sick, or you undergo a level of illness somewhere in between. Covid aside, for those of you who travel by airplane, here is a great way to evaluate your immune system. Do you fall ill or catch a cold or catch something else after a plane trip? Those of you who do are most likely suffering from a weakened immune system. There are products out now that you can take before and after you fly which help to boost your immune system with a goal of not "catching" anything. If your immune system is pretty strong anyway and you take these immune system boosters, it is very possible you will not get sick. If, however, you take these boosters and you still get sick, you may want to take a look at strengthening your immune system.

Most commonly, immune systems weaken when we deprive the body of the nutrients it needs to keep those cells strong. The quality and choices of the foods you eat help to determine the quality of the immune system you have. The efficiency of the human body was made to react to the quality (or lack thereof) of the nutrients we ingest. Proper nutrients keep us strong and healthy.

So, chances are, if we are not strong and healthy, then what we are eating is not providing the quality of nutrients we need to keep our immune system strong and healthy. And if the mind determines what we eat...

It is very easy to fall victim to illness. The new science of epigenetics suggests that only 10% of disease is genetic. The other 90% is from the environment we live in and the habits we maintain. I am not suggesting that all illness is our own fault. However, I am suggesting that we can take a more positive role in our own health. We can choose not to become a victim to whatever germs happen to get into our personal space by taking a more proactive role in our diet. We can choose our foods more wisely so that our immune system can stay as vigilant as it is capable of being. We can choose to manage our stress on a regular basis so that it does not create a debilitating disease. We can eat organic foods and use non-toxic cleaning products in the home to protect our immune systems. And we can clean out our bathroom cupboards and replace our personal care products with safer alternatives. All these options are available to us!

One strong reason to avoid getting sick is so you won't have to take antibiotics. When you ingest an antibiotic, as discussed in Chapter 9, *You Are What You Eat*, you kill off all those good bacteria, along with the bad. Ironically, this leaves you vulnerable to more disease! Your body is desperately trying to regenerate the good bacteria that have been killed off so that all affected systems can function normally again. Remember, one round of antibiotics kills off significant good bacteria which can take over six months to re-grow (in a healthy person), compromising your immune system even more as the regeneration is taking place.[54]

A helpful suggestion for when you do take an antibiotic is to take a round of probiotics, and maybe even prebiotics, afterwards (or, have a continuous regimen of both forms, if that is appropriate for your body). Pro- and prebiotics are helpful in rebuilding a healthy immune system and digestive system, but they are not the key to regenerating a healthy microbiome – that is determined by our food choices.

If you think about what antibiotics or other medications do to our bodies – degeneration and restoration – doesn't it make you wonder if most of this is even necessary? Could most of this be avoided if we chose to eat the healthiest of foods and managed our stress in a proactive way, keeping our immune systems as strong as they can be day after day?

So, are you going to choose to be an advocate for your body, or will you fall victim to sickness after sickness and take more and more prescription medications made of substances completely foreign to your body?

What role in this mind-body partnership will you choose?

---

[54] *Science Daily*, University of Copenhagen Study: "The Composition of Gut Bacteria Almost Recovers After Antibiotics," Oct. 23, 2018

THE MIND-BODY CONTRACT

Most successful partnerships have a contract. In negotiating that contract, there is compromise on both sides. If you were to write out a contract with your body, what compromises you would deem fair? What compromises would your body ask for, if it could, to get you to make different choices? No partnership is one-sided and no partnership is meant to be to the detriment of either party. Both parties need to feel not only that they are getting what they want, but also that they are compromising fairly and equally. A contract should be fair, honest, and one which allows both parties to maintain their integrity while fulfilling the reason for the contract.

With that in mind, I have created a starter contract that you can draw up with your body. Though this idea may seem silly to you, please humor me. Take a minute or two and read it through. What things would you change in your relationship with your body? What things would your body like to change? Make those edits and you will have crafted a contract that uniquely represents your mind-body partnership. Try it. Give yourself an opportunity to step into your body's potential for better and ultimate health. At the same time, you will be honoring your dreams and desires for your physical future.

My Mind-Body Partnership Contract
Effective Dates: Today – Forever

By means of this contract, I commit to taking full responsibility for my role in this mind-body partnership with the common desire for a long and healthy life. The Death Age I have chosen is _____. (See Chapter 4, Motivation vs. Inspiration, and complete the Dreams and Desires Worksheet.)

- ➢ I commit to doing the very best I can to provide my body with the nutrients it needs to stay strong and healthy and to avoid and/or severely limit any food that is toxic or detrimental to my health.
- ➢ I commit to doing my best to drink a stabilizing level of water each day to maintain a stasis of hydration throughout my body.

- I commit to doing the very best I can to exercise so as to give back to my body, building up to one hour a day in physical self-care.
- I commit to incorporating a stretching program within my exercise program to maintain the best level of flexibility I can throughout my joints and muscles.
- I commit to getting 7 – 9 hours of sleep each night so that my cells stand a chance of regenerating into healthy new cells each day.
- I commit to meditating, building up to a minimum of 20 minutes or more each day, whether it consists of sitting in silence or walking in nature or meditating in the traditional way, recognizing that the purpose of meditation is to remove distractions and quiet the mind.
- I commit to eating the healthiest foods I can afford, continuously providing my body with the fuel it needs to regenerate the healthiest cells and perform at its peak level.
- I commit to listening more intuitively to my body and the signals it is giving me so that I can better understand what it is requesting and provide it with what it needs.

In exchange,

- I expect my body to perform all duties that I ask.
- I expect all systems to continue to provide me with the basic and complex functions they were meant to perform.
- If I fail to fulfill my responsibilities, I expect my body to respond in a positive, direct line of communication so that I can understand what it needs each day.

I commit to loving my body as it is committed to loving me.

_____   _____
              Signed   Date

(For a pdf copy of this contract, please visit www.fitnessafterfortyfive.com and request through the contact page.)

THE PERSONIFICATION OF YOUR BODY, *OR:* YOU HAVE A FRIEND IN YOU!

To help with the concept of a partnership with your body, perhaps looking at it in a different way will allow you to wrap your arms around it, so to speak.

When I first started down the healthy road, my biggest obstacle was changing some of my food habits. I could come up with any excuse to "allow" myself a treat! As I learned more about ingredients and what they could do to my body, based on scientific evidence, it made my guilt shoot through the roof when I did "cheat." Now it wasn't just about eating food that wasn't on my diet, it was about eating food that actually was harmful to my body. My addiction was so strong that even then, I could still skirt around the discipline.

One day, I created "Lucille." I like to think of Lucille as my body buddy – actually my body angel – a personification of my body that stands by my side at all times.

Whenever I wanted to break my diet, I would imagine Lucille standing next to me. I would look at her and ask myself if I would offer her this food to eat. Lucille was my angel, my guardian, my friend. Her well-being depended entirely on me, so there was no way I would subject her to food that would hurt her. Slowly but surely, I realized that if I couldn't offer Lucille the food I was considering, how could I feed it to myself?

I then began to bring Lucille with me for most of my regimen.

Would I ever suggest she skip her workout? Would I make her stay up two hours past her comfortable bedtime? Would I ever suggest she skip her meditation or eat that pecan pie á la mode??

When I thought of my body as another person, I became much more objective. It became difficult for me to waive my responsibilities and not do what I knew was right and healthy to do. It allowed me to step back and consider the ramifications.

In caring and being responsible for Lucille and her wellbeing, I was better able to take care of myself. I was able to be kinder to myself. I was able to put myself first in order to be more effective in caring for others and teaching others about self-care. After all, we are all the primary caretakers of ourselves and our bodies, are we not? Our body depends on us to take that responsibility and do the best we can with it. In a sense, our bodies are our babies – completely dependent on our every decision to do the best for them and nurture them with the utmost care and to the best of our abilities.

This evolution for me took time – it took a long time. There were many habits to be broken, many new things to learn. To change the way I thought about and behaved towards myself was a huge shift. I had lived a certain way for forty-five years, with a multitude of habits and ways of doing things. When I started working with clients, I had to be sure the techniques that would help them with their new habits had been used successfully by me first. That was the only way I could be authentic and teach with integrity!

I also realized that it was okay to take a while to succeed. After all, if this were for the rest of my life, what was the hurry? One of the most helpful, influential thoughts I had was this: if there is a true bond and partnership between me and my body, and if the messages I was sending were of support and caring with matching behavior, what was I telling my body when I wasn't doing the best I could? What was the message I was telling it when I ate bad food or skipped a workout or two or three? Was the self-indulgence on my part worth the suffering I was inflicting on my body? How could my body possibly think that we were on the same side when I was self-sabotaging? I remember self-help author Louise Hay saying "your body is a mirror of your inner thoughts and beliefs." Was I giving as much as I could to have that body be as healthy as it could be? Was/Am I behaving in the most beneficial way that I can for my present and future health? Was/Am I living up to my side of the partnership?

And that is my daily mantra: Today I will make the best choices for myself and my body.

I am still not perfect. I do not think anyone reaches perfection. But I am very conscientious 99.9% of the time. When I do go "off course," my body is the first to let me know. The physical reaction it has when I go "off contract" is rather extraordinary, to the point that sometimes I laugh, realizing I did this to myself and it is my own darn fault! As with any partnership, there are instances of miscommunication and breaking the contract. However, by recognizing the critical relationship that the mind and the body have with each other, I have been able to create a much more compassionate understanding and attitude towards my body, not to mention a huge respect for all that it does for me and its ability to be ever ready upon my command.

I am proud to say, my mind-body partnership is a great success!

CHAPTER 10 RECAP

1) The body communicates with you all day long, but are you listening?
2) The body is a complex interconnected series of systems that communicate and interact with each other all day long. The multitude of functions that are going on behind the scenes all day, every day, are a marvel which should be admired and appreciated.
3) Our brain is in charge of how we move our bodies and what we feed our bodies. Our body has no power over the mind. What is your role in this mind-body partnership and how can you play your part in the best possible way?
4) When the body has an ache or a pain or a physical reaction to food or nature, do you react with respect and avoid that trigger in the future? Or do you continue to have the same reaction from repeated behavior and simply take a pill?
5) Pre- and post-menopause can take as long as 10 years for the entire cycle to proceed from beginning to the end. Respecting your body through this complex, inevitable process can be difficult.
6) Self-image and the aging body can take its toll on us psychologically. It's important to recognize what the body can do rather than what it can't.
7) You can choose to either be a victim to whatever befalls your physicality or you can be an advocate and do the best you can to prepare your body for whatever might happen to it.
8) Perhaps making a contract between your body and your mind will help solidify your commitment to take the utmost care of both.
9) Personifying your body as your friend may help you to gain a different perspective and respect for how you treat it.
10) The relationship between your mind and your body has a great influence on your future health and how you age.

Chapter 11

I. A.M. H.E.R.E.
THE SEVEN STEPS TO CONTROLLING YOUR PHYSICAL FUTURE

"You can't go back and change the beginning, but you can start where you are and change the ending."

C.S. Lewis

I. A.M. H.E.R.E. is an acronym that has a double meaning.

Its overall meaning is that you are being given just about everything you need to maintain a healthy lifestyle for the rest of your life. In addition, each of these seven letters is a foundation – a pillar – to put you in control of your aging well into your eighties and nineties. By choosing to master these, you will ideally be healthier and live a more active, engaged quality of life for decades to come.

When you think about the phrase, "I am here," you probably think of announcing yourself upon arriving at your destination, maybe even in a sing-song manner… "Yooo-hooo, I am here!"

"I am here" can also be a statement that suggests a starting-off point and implies that soon you are going somewhere else.

I would like to suggest that as you read through this section, you consider it as both: the place you are now (and I welcome you!) and also your position venturing forth with a new perspective, entering into a new way of life. The steps you will be taking are designed for your complete success.

The pillars these letters represent are:

> I = Immune System
> A = AHA! – Your Inspiration
> M = Meditation
> H = Hydration
> E = Exercise
> R = Rest
> E = Eating

Before we discuss these pillars, I would like you to join me in a meditation.

Don't worry if you have not meditated before, it is really simple to do. Read the meditation below and I know you will be able to do this immediately.

Let's begin!

Sit quietly in a comfortable chair. Place your feet firmly on the floor, knees bent and sitting up straight, with your back off the back of the chair. Place your hands gently on top of your thighs, palms up or down, whichever is more comfortable. Take a deep breath in and release it out. Take more long deep breaths and get yourself present in the room. Feel yourself relax with each breath and feel yourself present in the chair.

You are about to begin a full body scan, beginning with your toes, the bottoms of your feet, then the tops of your feet, your ankles and so on, one at a time. You will go from body part to body part, joint to joint, up your entire body including your shins, calves, knees, thighs front, thighs back, hips, buttocks, lower abdomen, upper abdomen, lower back, waist, sides of the torso, chest, upper back, shoulders, upper arms, elbows, forearms, wrists, hands and fingers, neck, and finally your head.

When you feel completely relaxed, begin to repeat the following phrase, "I sit in gratitude for my (name of body part). Up to this point in my life you have always done the best you could for me and I thank you. I am here now and moving forward."

It might seem like a lot, but practice makes perfect and soon you will be an ace at grounding yourself in gratitude. That is what this meditation is all about! Its purpose is to allow your mind to consider and thank each body part for all it has done for you over the years.

You can also do a shorter version of the meditation should you find that a particular body part needs some attention or is ailing. For instance, if you are suffering from allergies, say a prayer of gratitude for your lungs, your sinuses and your eyes. Thank them for all they have provided for you over the years. Apologize for the current ailment and say a healing prayer, always finishing in gratitude.

I have found that the more gratitude you show towards your body, the more aware you are of all it does. Your awareness piques your attention and you are much more inclined to be kind and cautious with all that you do.

Venturing forth on this journey, I suggest that you try to show your body the respect it deserves. Always remain grateful, giving your body more kindness, appreciation and thanks.

It is a true prerequisite to starting your "I am here" journey.

I - IMMUNE SYSTEM

Your number one focus for your future health and life should be your immune system.

A few theories as to why this is:

- The thymus gland tends to atrophy as we get older, promoting a decrease in T cells which results in a decrease in the ability to fight off infection.
- Bone marrow cells have become lazier and can no longer create the necessary stem cells that are needed to support the immune system.
- The older we get, the less attentive we are to what we eat, and the poorer the diet, the weaker the immune system.

Chances are, if an older person is exposed to a strange infection, he or she is not able to combat the new germs efficiently and is more inclined to get sick. However, having said that, "only a small percentage – let's say 10% - of the decline in immunity is caused by aging itself."[55]

How the Immune System Works

In a nutshell, when a diseased cell manifests in the body like a cancer cell or virus, the NK (Natural Killer) cells recognize it as bad and destroy it by puncturing holes in the cell's membrane and filling it with poisons that then kill it. The stronger your immune system, the faster it is able to perform this duty and keep ahead of the NK cells. (I just have to say that when I was reading about this, I was truly in awe at the body's efficiency in performing this task. How on earth does it know what to do? Fortunately for us, it does. I am incredibly grateful for this innate function of my immune system.)

It is the immune system that protects us from virtually every disease and malfunction the body can have. It is, therefore, of critical importance that you put your immune system at the top of your priority list.

So, how do you do that?

A healthy immune system is a result of the food you eat, the exercise you provide your body, the hydration level you keep, the rest you get,

---

[55] *AARP Bulletin*, September 2020

the mental clarity you maintain and the environment you choose. The immune system drives your train. The only way it can stay strong is for you to embrace your responsibility and fortify it by feeding yourself healthy non-toxic food, sleeping well (your body produces necessary fortifying proteins while you sleep), keeping a handle on your stress levels, exercising and partaking in all the other healthy habits we have mentioned and the new ones we will be addressing.

Taking supplements like vitamin C, echinacea or zinc is a good thing to do when your body is sick. If you are supplementing when your immune system doesn't need it, you are basically telling the immune system to lay low because the supplements will handle it. Your immune system stays strong by working and fighting off pathogens. That is its job. But when your immune system has been weakened by some sort of germ, that is the time for supplementation. There are quite a few supplements in addition to those mentioned that can support it and help it get strong and be successful at getting you back to good health.

It's All Connected: The Immune System, Inflammation and Disease

When a disease, virus, fungus, mold, germ, bad bacterium, parasite or other toxin invades the body, the immune system's sensors are triggered. In the battle against these "foreigners," cells of the immune system fight back and an inherent reaction occurs, created to destroy the pathogen and/or its environment. A by-product created with this protective attack is inflammation.

When inflammation occurs, blood circulation increases to the infected area. The blood vessels of the affected area actually dilate to help increase the blood flow. Through this process, the immune cells flow into the area helping to abate the infection. Ideally, in due time, the infection or foreign substance causing the imbalance disappears and is healed.

But what if there is no infection? What if the inflammation is there due to poor diet, lack of sleep, toxins ingested through the air, water and food, etc.? What if your body is in a constant state of inflammation without a specific pathogen? From all the inflammation with the immune system on high alert, white blood cells are continuously being pumped throughout your blood system and chemical messengers are maintaining that high level of defense 24 hours a day.

So, when the body is in a chronic state of inflammation, it disrupts the ability to interfere with pathogens and any outside toxin. Dr. Andrew Weil explains it this way, "Whole-body inflammation refers to chronic, imperceptible, low-level inflammation. Mounting evidence suggests that over time this kind of inflammation sets the foundation for many serious, age-related diseases including heart disease, cancer and neurodegenerative conditions such as Alzheimer's and Parkinson's diseases. Recent evidence indicates that whole-body inflammation may also contribute to psychological disorders, especially depression."[56]

If your diet is already one consisting of highly acidic foods, as mentioned in *You Are What You Eat*, then inflammation is already very comfortable existing inside of you, making this fight for the immune system much more difficult to win.

One of the biggest weakening forces of our immune system is sugar. A 12-ounce can of Coke, as an example, has 39 grams of sugar, which is almost ¼ cup!! And, due to their high sugar density, most soda beverages are highly acidic. It's that high concentration of acidity that creates the inflammation that weakens the immune system.

Another main source that weakens our immune system is stress. According to the American Psychological Association, based on almost 300 studies done by Suzanne Segerstrom, PhD, of the University of Kentucky, and Gregory Miller, PhD, of the University of British Columbia, "For stress of any significant duration - from a few days to a few months or years, as happens in real life - all aspects of immunity went downhill. Thus, long-term or chronic stress, through too much wear and tear, can ravage the immune system."[57]

---

[56] drweil.com/diet-nutrition/anti-inflammatory-diet-pyramid, "Reducing Whole Body Inflammation?"

[57] apa.org (American Psychological Association), Psychological Science/Research in Action, "Stress Weakens the Immune System"

The University of Virginia Center for Brain Immunology and Glia is studying and researching the connection between the brain and the immune system. Though it is said to be too soon to identify precisely *how* the two systems are connected, a healthy immune system could offset potential issues with the brain, such as Alzheimer's and dementia, Parkinson's, Multiple Sclerosis, Autism Spectrum Disorder and Depression.[58]

It is not just the brain that is affected by an unhealthy immune system. Most heart disease is a result of inflammation, which can be triggered by a weak immune system. An unhealthy immune system is also being attributed to some cancers. "The immune system is our natural first line of defense against cancer."[59] Thus, building and maintaining a strong immune system should be the cornerstone of a good cancer-fighting and cancer-preventing foundation.

Ironically, the healthier your immune system, the less aware you are of any of this even happening. In many instances, it all goes on without your knowledge or without any noticeable reaction by your body. You simply go about your day-to-day life while your immune system fights to maintain homeostasis, or balance.

Think of it like this. Two people are exposed at the same time to someone with a cold or the flu. One of them gets sick but the other does not. This has everything to do with the strength of their individual immune systems.

Keep in mind that millions of cells, in our immune system and throughout our body, die every day and are replaced with new cells. Seeing that these new cells are created from within, it makes sense to suggest that the quality of these new cells is determined by the condition and health of our body and mind. The condition and health of our body and mind are based not only on the fuel we ingest and the behaviors we choose, but also on the toxins that surround us. All these factors work in sync to either support the immune system or weaken it.

---

[58] med.virginia.edu/big/
[59] thetruthaboutcancer.com, "Understanding Your Immune System and Cancer" (video)

My suggestion is to take control of what you can to support your immune system so that it can serve you positively and help stave off whatever potential diseases might be lurking.

A Word about Autoimmune Diseases

I am sure, by now, that you are familiar with the term, "autoimmune." The typical definition is that the body's immune system is attacking itself. This is not quite the case. What is taking place is that the immune system is reacting to various toxins in the body either from diet (which comes from the pesticides, herbicides, or insecticides used in food), pollution of water or air, heavy metals, reaction to pharmaceuticals, and even the chemicals the body creates from stress. Basically, the immune system is responding to that which it recognizes as doing harm, and is making an effort to right itself. A state of chronic inflammation is present and the immune system is overworked.

Autoimmune diseases can run in families and there is much research being done to study the genetics involved. "Although genetics play a key role in autoimmune risk, environmental factors are known to have a large impact on the emergence of autoimmune conditions."[60] So, your mother and grandmother having lupus means that you may be prone to it, but *your* environmental factors, over which you mostly have control, are up to you. You do not have to get lupus, too.

Over 100 autoimmune disorders have been identified, the most recognized being: rheumatoid arthritis, lupus, chronic fatigue syndrome, fibromyalgia, Addison's disease, celiac disease, multiple sclerosis, Hashimoto's thyroiditis, Crohn's disease, Guillain-Barre, psoriasis, and the list goes on.

To avoid this horrific journey, do all the suggestions that are written in this book. But, most importantly, listen to your body and what it is trying to tell you. Don't ignore the symptoms. And because of the myriad of possible

---

[60] ifm.org/news-insights (Institute for Functional Medicine), "Genetic Predisposition in Autoimmune Disease & Emerging Research"

diseases, it might help to do your own research alongside your doctor's; it could shorten a possible 7-14 year average that it can take for a diagnosis.

A – AHA!

If your purpose for reading this book is to change your life and give your body a fair chance at aging healthily, and you haven't yet completed the *Motivation vs. Inspiration* chapter's Dreams and Desires Worksheet, I invite you to mark your place here and go do that now. Your "AHA!" is pretty well covered in that chapter.

The worksheet is important because it gets you to really think about the decades you have lived and how you want to live the rest of your life. We do not typically think about our future in the way the worksheet asks us to, nor do we anticipate what our physicality will *need* to be in order to live the way we want and hope to live. I do not want to give away any of the basics of the worksheet if you haven't done it… so, please pause now, go back to Chapter 4 and answer the questions as instructed.

The key takeaway from this task is to recognize that change is hard. But change that is from the heart and not the head is change that has a much better chance of working. Being inspired to change gets to you through emotion and emotion will help you be faithful to your new behavior.

Keep in mind, and I am sure you will agree, the medical community can keep us alive into our 80s, 90s, even 100s – but can those medical personnel keep us alive living the quality of life we want, or is their primary concern longevity? The "AHA!" lies not in the quantity of life, but in the quality. And it is the choices you make today that will determine the quality of your life in the decades to come.

These choices and changes do not need to be made all at once. Like the mountain climber preparing for Everest, a slower, gradual, step-by-step transition is best. As you lose the bad habits and define new good ones, your body will be very aware of your intentions and level of commitment. When the body knows you are trying, it is much more inclined to support you and help you to succeed. And, who knows – perhaps you will want to change that worksheet after a decade or two and create more "AHAs" for your future.

M – MEDITATION

We started this chapter off with a meditation. How did it go? Did you feel a difference in both your mind and your relaxation? Is meditation new for you or have you practiced it before?

Though it may not seem to be this way, meditation is actually one of the most important steps you can take in embracing a healthy aging process and an overall healthy life. Meditation is the answer to a multitude of issues that can befall us as we age. There are more and more studies being done on the effects of meditation on our mental health, especially PTSD, depression and anxiety. Studies are also being done on the relationship between meditation and chronic pain, sleep disorders, diabetes, blood pressure, binge eating disorder, and a multitude of other detrimental physical issues. The bottom line is that even sitting quietly for 5 minutes per day helps to calm our minds and slow our bodies down, which ultimately affects our stress levels and our overall health.

Meditation can take place in many different formats. Gone are the days of believing we have to find a mosque with a large gong, wear all white and sit cross-legged on the floor in order to meditate.

There is **metta meditation** which is sending positive energy to others through a repetition of mantras.

There is **Transcendental Meditation** (TM) where you are taught by a certified instructor who customizes a practice for you. You learn a mantra for you and you alone that you repeat over and over for your meditation.

There is **chakra meditation** where you focus on the energy centers of the body, one at a time.

There is **guided meditation** where you listen to someone speak and guide you on a meditative journey.

There is **movement meditation** where you move your body in gentle ways with full focus on your body in relationship to the movement.

There is a **body scan relaxation meditation** where you are typically reclined and begin by focusing on your toes then slowly go body part by body part up the body as you relax each stop along the way until your entire body is in a completely relaxed state.

There is **mindfulness meditation** where you are totally focused on what it is you are doing. Eating mindfully is popular, where you focus on each and every bite (and even chew) you take while you eat. I have been in a mindfulness class where we took one raisin and chewed on it for 10 minutes, focusing on every sensation it offered with each chew. Even sitting quietly in a chair looking out the window and watching every single thing that happens out that window is a mindfulness meditation. The object is to be totally present with whatever it is that you are focusing on.

There is **spiritual meditation** where you may pray to a higher power either from your religious practice or your own form of spirituality, bringing yourself closer to that entity.

There is **focused meditation** where you find something to focus on, be it your breath, a candle flame, mala beads, music, the sound of gongs — anything that will be supportive of your focus. Mala beads helped me when I first started meditating and I still enjoy using them, especially when I travel.

Deep breathing or diaphragmatic breathing meditation is when you don't just focus on your breath, but you inhale with the full distention of the diaphragm and exhale with the complete emptying of the lungs. This is my preferred choice of meditation at this time of my life. I follow the advice of David Ji, a world-renowned meditation teacher, which is "RPM": Rise, Pee, Meditate. That way, my day doesn't begin until I meditate. This practice has helped me the most.

Whatever modality you choose, simply sitting quietly and focusing on your breath is meditation. It is important to start out with deep inhales and exhales. That will help your body to relax, then you can breathe normally. You do not have to empty your mind – although many find it much nicer if they imagine being near a waterfall, on a beach, in a forest or on top of a mountain to provide that extra sense of calm before they begin. I am fortunate that I live near the ocean and can choose to sit and stare out my window at the sea, or go to a different window and look at the leaves on the trees blowing or changing colors in the fall, or go to another window and look at the intricacies of the stone walls that surround my yard. I can just as easily choose a picture in the house to look at. Even better is to venture outside and become one with nature. Stealing snippets of meditation throughout the day helps you to refocus on you and your well-being. You will be surprised how quickly the time goes and how relaxed you become.

For the body's sake, meditate for at least five minutes each day. Ideally you should work up to twenty minutes a day, but even if you just have five or ten minutes at a time, the benefits will still appear. And when you get into the habit you will find you do not have to focus on your breathing any longer – it will happen naturally. The most important component of meditation is to be present every moment. Focus on exactly where you are and what you have chosen to look at or imagine.

If you are one who sits at a desk much of the day, please do not meditate there. Get up and move to a quiet place, isolated from the phone, computer or distractions. I know people who actually use a bathroom for meditation, and I have a friend who uses a closet. As a matter of fact, in my FIT Workshop, I teach the practice of 55 + 5. When you work at a desk for extended periods of time, it is important to take a 5 minute break every 55 minutes – to stretch the body and distract the mind to help it better focus upon your return to your desk. By getting up, going to a window or picture in your home and take 2-3 minutes to be mindful, you will be amazed at how much better you will feel at the end of the day.

The main goal with doing a meditation is to be alone and in quiet. Start slowly and build up the amount of time you spend until you are comfortable being in quiet and peace for twenty minutes or more each session. Feel free to set a timer. If you are app savvy, there are quite a few of them you can use for meditation. Meditation applications vary – you can find an app that plays soothing music, or one that has guided meditations where a voice creates imagery for you or takes you on a journey, like we did at the beginning of this chapter. Choose whichever works best for you and experiment. You will quickly learn what you like and do not like! The important thing is to remember to be present with whatever practice you choose.

When you take this break from your stressors, you are giving your body and mind the gift of attention. You are recognizing that you do have stress, even though you may not feel it at the time. You are letting your body know you want to give back to it with gratitude for the many ways it supports you.

Always keep in mind that it is the effort that the body recognizes, not the perfection of the action you take. In other words, your body will react to your form of meditation and know that you are doing the best you can, no matter what format or modality you choose. As time goes by and your practice lengthens, your mind will be easier to quiet and you will find you look forward to these moments where it is just you and total peace.

H – HYDRATION

What do you believe these days about how much water you should drink? And do you only count water, or do you include other liquids, like soda? Coffee? Juice? Fruit?

How Much Water is Enough?

There are varying theories about how much water is enough. There are as many answers as there are people, because everyone is different.

One standard of measurement reports you should drink, in ounces, the number of kilograms you weigh. In America, this means we divide your weight by 2.2. This can become very unrealistic if you are carrying too many extra pounds.

Another standard of measurement calls for eight 8-ounce glasses of water each and every day – this certainly keeps it simple, but it may not be the right amount for many people.

When I ask my clients how much water they drink, most will tell me they drink plenty! But when I ask them to actually measure how much they are drinking, there is a moment of truth and they see that "plenty" is about half of what it needs to be.

Here is an easy way to help you keep track of your daily water intake. In the morning, line up your water bottles or glasses and keep them in an obvious and convenient place. Because they are visible, you will be reminded about your water intake every time you see your daily lineup. And you'll get a visual sense of where you stand in terms of rationing your intake throughout the day. For instance, I use four 16 ounce bottles as my minimum each day. I try to finish the first bottle by 9:00am, second by 12:00noon, third by 3:00pm and the last one by dinner. This is a great way for you to determine that you are, in fact, drinking "enough."

Here's a good test to determine if you are getting the hydration you need: What color is your urine?

If your urine is dark yellow, you most likely are not hydrated enough. If the color of your urine is a pale yellow, you are probably fine. If the color is so light that you can barely see a yellow tone, you are most likely drinking too much water and cutting back a bit would be in your best interest. Perhaps, spread out your ingestion more. And, as always, if you see any discoloration that persists, you might want to give a call to your doctor. Better safe than sorry. (Do keep in mind that some supplements and prescription drugs contribute to urine color, so do your research based on what you are taking.)

Water begins to be absorbed in your system as soon as it hits your mouth. If you are underhydrated, though, and need to absorb liquid quickly, keep in mind that "if there are carbohydrates and electrolytes in a drink, it increases the rate of fluid absorption."[61]

And why on earth do we even need so much water?

In a word, hydration. Monitoring your hydration is one of the most critical voluntary actions you can take to maintain your health every day for the rest of your life. Maintaining a steady level of hydration helps keep your body temperature stable, offsets muscle stiffness, helps with blood pressure regulation, participates in the body's waste disposal system and assists in the transport of nutrients and oxygen throughout the body. Keeping a steady level of hydration as you age eases the aging process and offsets a plethora of potential issues.

Here are some interesting facts that might surprise you:

- Second only to air, water (hydration) is needed to sustain life. Your body is made up of approximately 65% water spread throughout your organs, tissues and systems. Muscle tissue alone is 70-75% water. Imagine how more supple and flexible your muscles would be with enough hydration.[62]
- You should beware of the high levels of caffeine in energy drinks. The latest scientific research has shown that a cup or two of coffee does not have the dehydrating effect as originally believed. *However*, these new versions of "caffeine-in-a-bottle" drinks are extremely high in caffeine levels, causing dehydration, depending on how many are consumed in a day.[63] A good rule of thumb if you are drinking these beverages is to drink additional glasses of water along with them!
- Soda has very high levels of sodium (we already discussed the high levels of sugar), so you need to make sure it does not offset your natural levels of sodium. In other words, if ingesting high concentrations of sodium, you may want to drink several more

---

[61] *American Council on Exercise Pro Source,* April 2016
[62] *ACE Fitness Matters,* July/August 2007
[63] *The World's Healthiest Foods,* June 2017

glasses of water to balance the increase in your sodium intake from the soda.

- Water comes in all kinds of food. Fruits and vegetables are comprised of 70%-99% water. Meat comes in at approximately 50%-60% water, pasta between 60% – 69% water and bread can contribute as much as 39% water.[64] So next time you are "hungry," it could be your body signaling its desperation to get something to drink! (Beware, though, that some simple carbohydrates like crackers, chips and cookies have less than 10% water!) For those of you watching your weight, when you sense hunger, drink a full glass of water, wait 20 minutes, and if you are still hungry then have something nutritious to eat.
- Thirst is a sign that the body has already begun dehydration. The sensation of thirst dissipates the older you are. People in their 80s rarely feel thirsty. If you are in that age bracket or know someone who is, thinking that "your body will let you know" could be very misleading. If an elderly person admits to being "thirsty," they are most likely already dehydrated. (As my mother moved into her 90s, she had several 3- to 5-day hospital visits simply from dehydration.) If you maintain a steady hydration level throughout the day, then you will very likely never feel thirsty. For those who live in a warmer climate or have a summer season and you tend to perspire throughout the day, you need to monitor your hydration.
- Your brain is 75% water[65] – need I say more? Something to think about if you have persistent headaches, foggy brain or dizziness.
- "When people dehydrate 3 percent of their body weight (for example, you weigh 100 pounds and you lose three pounds of water), there's about a 2 percent decline in calorie burning per day." [66] For those of you trying to lose weight, this is not a good thing! Weight loss is regulated by the speed of your body's

---

[64] nih.org (National Institutes of Health), US National Library of Medicine, "Water, Hydration and Health," August 2010

[65] usgs.gov (United States Government Science), Water Science School, "The Water in You: Water and the Human Body," May 22, 2019

[66] healthcare.utah.edu (University of Utah), "Is Eight Enough? Dr. Wayne Askew Hydration Study," January 14, 2003

- metabolism (the rate at which your body burns calories) and this determines how fast you lose weight as well. Again, maintaining a steady hydration level keeps your metabolism functioning at its peak performance level.
- Just a slight dip in your overall hydration can make you sleepy and make it difficult to concentrate. This is of particular concern if you will be driving any length of time. To be smart, before you start a long ride, build up your hydration level and keep it steady throughout the trip. Yes, you might have to make bathroom stops along the way, but getting out of the car and stretching your legs is not such a bad thing! Think of your hydration maintenance as your flexibility enhancer!
- Twenty-two percent of your bone tissue, believe it or not, is made up of water.[67] As we age, we have to consider that our bones become brittle and break more easily. Hydration is one way to support healthy bone tissue.
- Sports drinks are higher in sugar and lower in electrolytes than you probably think. If you drink sports drinks in an effort to replace electrolytes lost during exercise, please *read the label* first. One of the most popular sports drinks shows the first two ingredients as water, then high fructose corn syrup. After that it says the beverage contains less than 0.05% of the electrolytes and minerals you were drinking it for! Sports drinks are for serious athletes and people who have strenuous jobs in the outdoors who sweat a lot. They are most certainly not a recreational beverage. And when you calculate the amount of sugar in them, you won't want to drink them anyway!

Dehydration

Remember, not enough water in your system sets off an imbalance in your sodium levels which can be evident through dizziness, cramping, drops in blood pressure and many other symptoms.

---

[67] usgs.gov, (United States Government Science), Water Science School, "The Water in You: Water and the Human Body," May 22, 2019

Signs of ongoing or chronic dehydration include constipation, headaches, high blood pressure, fatigue, spontaneous muscle cramping, asthma and allergies, high cholesterol, bladder and/or kidney problems, skin disorders, digestive issues, joint pain and stiffness, and weight gain.[68] If any of these symptoms continue to appear in your life, be serious about checking your water intake.

Are you aware that many elderly people have been diagnosed with dementia and it has simply been a case of dehydration? If you are a caretaker or notice someone you see on a regular basis showing signs of mental fogginess, it could simply be dehydration.

Staying hydrated should be a daily habit and is well worth the effort. Chronic dehydration has been proven to be the cause of many chronic conditions. So, when you make the decision to focus on hydration and achieve stable levels, you may discover that issues you are dealing with simply disappear. I am not saying they will, but hydration plays an important role – so, you never know until you try.

E – EXERCISE

You have heard it before, exercise is a key ingredient to a healthy life. Study after study has shown that an exercise regimen each week can help to offset cancer of all kinds, heart disease, hypertension (high blood pressure), type 2 diabetes, osteoporosis, arthritis, joint issues ... the list goes on and on. A regular exercise program enhances your quality of life tenfold!

Various chapters in this book -- *Exercise Is A Gift, BodSpir® Meditative Strength Training, Flexibility is the Key* and *The Forgotten Muscle* -- all detail pretty much everything you need to know about exercise. But here are just a few other ideas to add to the repertoire.

Many of the issues we attribute to aging should be blamed on the real culprit: misuse of our bodies and lack of care. There is a recurring theme

---

[68] waterbenefitshealth.com, "Twelve Symptoms of Chronic Dehydration"

found in scientific studies on aging that shows if you want to extend your life span and stay healthy, you need to maintain a regular exercise program.

A regular exercise program has been defined by the American College of Sports Medicine, the leading authority on exercise, as 150 minutes of moderate-intensity exercise per week and two-to-three sessions of strength training a week. Not only is exercise good for the body, but there is increasing evidence suggesting that regular workouts protect and sharpen your mind, reduce stress and ward off depression and other mental illnesses.

As we age, we lose muscle tissue. Starting around age 30, we lose ½ pound of muscle per year. That is 15 pounds of muscle mass lost by the time you are 60! More often than not, those 15 pounds have been replaced with fat, because with loss of muscle comes a lessening of metabolism. However, when you are working your muscles and building muscle tissue (actually replenishing muscle tissue) it enhances your ability to burn calories. You are, in fact, changing your metabolism in a good way. As your muscle tissue maintains its strength and tone, your metabolism maintains its efficiency. This is one of the reasons why it is so important to include strength training as part of your exercise regime when you are over the age of forty-five.

As mentioned in the *Exercise is a Gift* chapter, the basis of all exercise is strength training. Get your body strong first. Once your muscles are strong and sturdy, you can do just about anything you want with little-to-no risk, provided you have trained properly. I have long thought this was the case, but then I actually lived it.

A couple of years ago, I had the very fortunate opportunity to take a month off from my normal life. I moved out to the west coast and lived in my daughter's apartment. The first thing I did, as I did not have a car, was walk all around her neighborhood to look for a gym where I could work out. What I found was a Pilates studio. I had never really done Pilates before, so this would be a perfect chance for me to learn this exercise regimen. As an added bonus, they offered variations: TRX, springboard, mat, as well as private Pilates sessions and different yoga classes. It was perfect.

I started right in and typically did a variety of classes four or five times each week for the four weeks I was there. Each class had a unique offering and I loved all of them. Great instructors, great students, great experience. When I got home and started into my regular strength training program, I was surprised that I could not comfortably lift the weights I was lifting before. I was actually weaker than I was before I left! Wanting to be able to quantify my discovery, over the next few sessions, I did the exercises I used to do and saw what weight I could use to get the same level of exertion for each specific exercise. Long story short, I discovered that I had lost 22% of my strength – that was after 4 weeks of 4 or 5 classes each week of yoga or Pilates. Bottom line: Do strength training above all other forms of exercise! Twice a week is sufficient. Then do all other forms of exercise the rest of the week. And mix it up. Your body will love the challenge!

Regardless of which exercise regimen you choose, it is crucial that you maintain this mindset: The sole purpose of exercise is to give back to your body. Setting that intention allows the body to focus on all the benefits it is receiving from the exercise so it doesn't have to think about anything else but receiving those benefits.

As previously mentioned, another critical aspect of maintaining good physical conditioning is flexibility. I designed BodSpir® with this in mind. Stretching is incorporated throughout each workout, which helps offset the muscle contractions you are doing with each strengthening exercise.

One last note about exercise - if you are the type who finds accountability important, find a friend or a class. If you are unsure about what to choose, find a personal trainer, but make sure they are experienced with someone your age and know how to work with your current exercise ability. Remember, if you don't like what they are telling you to do, let them know. Communication is the most important component between a trainer and a client.

The key to a successful exercise program is to participate in something that you actually enjoy doing. (I am the first to admit that strength training is not necessarily something that you will enjoy doing. I don't enjoy it either!! BodSpir® does make it easier.) By choosing something that will also challenge you means you are bound to see improvement. You also want variety and the ability to enhance your body's functioning through several different approaches.

And I cannot emphasize this enough – find an exercise regimen that works for YOU. The bottom line is to just do it. The rewards will be given back to you with as much enthusiasm as you put into it.

R – REST

Let's chat about sleep. We all need it, some more than others. One thing for sure is that we can't live without it. Although we feel nothing, our body is very busy restoring all the "damage" we did the day before, as well as some new creations. During sleep, our body recovers from stress as well as helping with brain, muscle and organ tissue growth. Typically, our body temperature is a tad lower and our muscles relax while we sleep. We breathe deeper and slower. Our stomach is at rest and many cells die and get replenished. Our blood is dirtied by day and cleansed by night. Our brain, too, rids itself of toxins overnight. Our memories are also tagged and archived, so to speak. Our liver and gallbladder are busy assuring that all the toxins have been processed and our kidneys and intestines gear up to rid our body of them.

If we are sleeping "normally," about 8 hours, we alternate through 5 cycles of Rapid Eye Movement (REM) sleep and Non-Rapid Eye Movement (NREM) sleep, each cycle lasting approximately 90 minutes. Briefly, REM sleep, the deep sleep, is thought of as the dream stage of sleep – when our rational self lets go and anything is possible, which is why dreams can be so crazy. NREM sleep is about 75% of our sleep time and during its deepest stages the body takes care of all that repair work that needs to be done.

How Much Sleep Is Enough?

I could go on and on with all the scientific research on determining how much sleep we need and why. There are a lot of things to take into consideration: your Circadian Rhythm and the effect it has on your sleep cycle, suggested times to go to bed and to wake up, what happens if you have sleep apnea, which is the best mattress, the best pillow....

The bottom line is this: Are you getting enough sleep? Before you answer that, it may be interesting to look at your sleep history to see if you have *ever* gotten enough sleep. To help you with that, I want to share a bit of my sleep story and how it has changed over the years.

In my twenties, living in New York City, I awoke at 7:00am, showered, ate and set out to walk to work (a New York thing!) arriving by 9:00am raring to go! I left work between 5:00 and 6:00pm, and most nights stopped to meet someone for cocktails. A few drinks later, a bite to eat and it would be time to cab it home, and I would fall into bed around midnight. Seven hours later, I would wake up and do the whole thing over again. Nothing interfered with sleep. Not even the alcohol.

In my late twenties to early thirties I was traveling all over the world and often didn't even know which time zone I was in. With my job, I would sometimes get 4 hours of sleep, other nights maybe 8. Sometimes the only sleep I got was on an airplane! But it didn't seem to matter. When it was time to get up and go, I got up and went!

As I moved into my mid-thirties, there was a definite shift. I felt the need for more sleep, whether I was able to get it or not. Then after the arrival of the children, forget about it. There was never enough sleep and I really suffered because of it. Erratic sleep meant an erratic metabolism and it was very difficult to lose the weight I had gained from pregnancy.

In my forties, with the kids now older and maintaining their own sleep patterns, I was able to develop mine and find a rhythm. This was also the time in life I took a deep look at my overall health and became interested in the fitness industry as a career. Because of that, it made sense to support my interest in improved health with better sleep, and this I did.

I paid more attention to both the time I awoke and the time I went to bed. While the kids were in school, we all got up very early, and this meant we also all went to bed at a reasonable hour, too, or were at least in our rooms with the doors closed.

As my fifties arrived and the kids were driving and on their own to get themselves up and out for the day, I was able to really get into my own rhythm based on my life and my responsibilities. Regarding sleep, I did not have any other responsibilities, except to myself.

Life has pretty much remained that way as I move forward into my seventies.

I am a morning person. I do better when I get up by 5:30am and go to bed no later than 9:30pm. I head off to bed at 9:00pm, and I gift myself a half-hour of reading to ease myself into a relaxed state.

I rarely wake up in the middle of the night, which means I usually sleep a good solid 7½-8 hours each night. Every now and then I have that rough night where I do wake up and I can't get back to sleep – my brain is running a mile a minute and it won't stop. When that happens, I get up, go downstairs and make myself a cup of chamomile tea. I usually turn on a Harry Potter movie, sipping and emptying my brain instead of revving it up with thought. Shortly thereafter, I return to bed and I'm able to immediately go back to sleep. This can take up to an hour.

Now, let's move on to you. How have your sleep patterns developed or changed over the years? How does that history influence your current sleep habits? What time do you awaken and go to bed? Are you a middle-of-the-night bathroom tripper, and can you get right back to sleep if you are?

As you move through your decades, how did your sleep patterns relate to your life at the time? How do your sleep patterns relate to your life now? Is there anything really standing in the way of you rightly claiming a good night's sleep? And, if so, what can you do to be kinder to yourself and more respectful of what your body needs?

If you are feeling sleep deprived, it is very important that you address it. According to the Centers for Disease Control, sleep deprivation is defined as getting fewer than 7 hours per night over an extended period of time. Doing that for years on end is definitely a cause for concern. There are myriad issues that can arise due to lack of sleep or inconsistent sleep patterns.

You might have memory lapses or difficulty concentrating.

You could experience drowsiness while driving which is something to be really concerned about. (Each year, drowsy driving accounts for about 100,000 crashes, 71,000 injuries, and 1,550 fatalities, according to the National Safety Council. Drowsy driving contributes to an estimated 9.5% of all crashes, according to AAA.)

Sleep deprivation can be directly related to a weakened immune system, leading to frequent colds and infections.

You could have difficulty coping with stress. (Chapter 12, *Stress: The Silent Saboteur*, will go into more detail on alleviating this.)

You might find you are moodier or more quick-tempered than usual. Our animalistic switch is more easily activated making us more irrational.

You might experience weight gain or a lower sex drive – which, assuming you are at least in your 40's, is compounded with menopause.

Sleep issues can result in higher rates of depression and anxiety.

You might find it difficult to concentrate or feel like you have a "foggy" brain.

There is an increased risk of diabetes, disruption in hormone function, increased risk of a heart attack and an overall lack of motivation.

Obviously, it really is important to get adequate sleep each and every night.

Here are some ideas if you do suffer from sleep deprivation:

- Finish eating and drinking alcohol at least 2 to 3 hours before bed.
- Do not use your computer or any handheld device at least 30 to 60 minutes before bedtime and do not keep them in your bedroom. If you must be in the same room, turn the computer off, or close the laptop. And turn your phone so the screen is face down.
- If you are a caffeine drinker, have your last drink at least 6 hours before bed.
- Add a small amount of fermented food to your diet, like Kombucha Tea (4 ounces, 2 to 3 times/day,) or ¼ cup of sauerkraut.
- Make sure your bed is only for sleep and intimacy – do not bring work to bed with you.
- If you wake up in the middle of the night, try not to look at the clock. (For me, this one helped tremendously!)
- If you read or watch TV before bed, avoid indulging in violence or tension – or the news!
- Create a bedtime ritual at the same time every evening.
- Make sure the room temperature is comfortable.
- Make sure the bed is comfortable.
- Check any medications you take for possible side effects regarding sleep.
- If not asleep in 15-20 minutes, get up, go to another room to read or listen to soft music or meditate, then try again when drowsy.
- Maintain a healthy diet (preferably plant-based) and exercise regularly.
- Sadly enough, it could be your pets in bed with you that disrupts your sleep, and that might have to change.

Napping

How could we leave the discussion of *rest* without discussing napping? Never shy away from napping. A quick 20-30 minute nap in the middle of the afternoon can often revive you for the rest of the day. If you have traveled to other countries, you are aware that people in many countries take "siestas," or afternoon breaks. It is a definite way to recharge. If, however, you find that you need to 'nap' longer than a half hour, it might be best to check with some of the other possible issues already mentioned.

Beware if the nap is taken too late in the afternoon. This could interrupt that night's sleep and throw your system all out of whack. Simply be conscious about it.

An alternative to a nap in the afternoon is to meditate. Taking twenty minutes to sit quietly and relax can be extremely re-energizing. You don't even have to go into a deep, empty-the-brain kind of meditation. Simply sit quietly in a chair and look out the window. Let the thoughts come and go, provided they aren't stressful. Try being present with whatever you are seeing out the window and stay with it. The tension in your body will begin to subside and you will feel a recharge sure to take you through until bedtime. Of course, I recommend meditation in the afternoon whether you need a rest or not because it is a great gift to give yourself each day!

Sleeping well at night has everything to do with your behavior during the day. Therefore, if you follow all the other suggestions you are learning in this book, a full night's sleep – every night – will come naturally.

E - EATING

As I have already shared with you, I have had food issues as long as I can remember. I believed I was overweight my entire life and I always thought I was bigger than I was. Along with this body dysmorphia, I was an occasional binge eater and a sugar addict. This evolved over time, getting stronger as I matured into adulthood. It all continued with me until I got into the fitness industry, and even then, my bad habits took years to kick.

The solution might seem so simple to most, but it was something that still took time to realize and accept. The magic key was education. When I started learning about what was in my food and consequently what I was putting in my body, it was a wake-up call.

The more I learned, the more it led me to accept the path of veganism and the decision to eat local organic as much as possible. I am fierce about eating organic foods when I am at home and, if at all possible, when not at home. This has been the best diet for me and I am grateful for the realization and the discovery.

The chapter *You Are What You Eat* pretty much covers the suggestions I would urge you to heed when venturing to create a healthier diet for yourself. Remember as you bully forth, you are not "going on a diet." You are changing how you eat to that which is healthier for you. I have to say, I have never understood dieting, per se – changing your eating habits to lose weight only to stop the "diet" and revert back to all your old eating habits. This is exactly what the vast majority of dieters do, and the outcome is always the same – the weight goes right back on!

Instead of "going on a diet," take a longer, proactive approach and change the foods you eat, make smarter choices and gradually stick to the new habits you develop. You don't have to worry about losing weight; it will come off on its own!

After struggling with my eating habits my entire life, it was only after I learned the things I shared with you in *You Are What You Eat* (and that is just the tip of the iceberg!) that I realized how to listen to my body, be kinder to my body, treat it with more respect and feed it only good, healthy foods so that it, in turn, can give me a healthier physical future.

There are several resources I use to keep updated with what is going on in the food industry. For your reference, my key resources regarding food are:

The Food Revolution.org	Environmental Working Group = ewg.org
Foodbabe.com	March-Against-Monsanto Facebook Group
Eatlocalgrown.com	Undergroundhealth.com
Althealthworks.com	Nongmoproject.org
Organicconsumers.org	Greenmedwellnesscenter.com

WRAPPING IT ALL UP!

When you think about it and are honest with yourself, the choices you make on a daily basis are yours and yours alone. For those things that are out of your control, allow them to be what they are and deal with them when the time is right. But for those choices that are yours, be brave and make the best ones you can at any given time.

Baby steps – one decision at a time, one choice at a time. And, when you start to make better choices for your body and your health, changes will begin to appear and you will slowly but surely begin to notice the vitality you are choosing to give to your body.

Remember always…

> *When you give to your body, your body will respond to you in kind.*

CHAPTER 11 RECAP

1) There are seven areas on which to focus to help gain a healthier lifestyle as you Thrive to 95. They create the acronym I. A.M. H.E.R.E.: I = Immune System, A = Aha! – Your Inspiration, M = Meditation, H = Hydration, E = Exercise, R = Rest, E = Eating.
2) A gratitude meditation can be done by sitting quietly and doing a full body scan, giving thanks for each body part as you progress through it.
3) A healthy immune system is a result of the food you eat, the exercise you provide to (and for) your body, the hydration level you keep, the rest you get, the mental clarity you maintain and the environment you choose. The immune system drives your train.
4) The choices you make today will determine the quality of your life for decades to come. When you discover your inspiration for life – your "aha" – you will be more inclined to make better choices.
5) There are more and more studies being done on the effects of meditation on our mental health, especially PTSD, depression and

anxiety. Studies are being done on the relationship between meditation and chronic pain, sleep disorders, diabetes, blood pressure, binge eating disorder, and a multitude of other detrimental physical issues. Even sitting quietly for 5 minutes per day helps to calm our minds and slow our bodies down, which ultimately affects our stress levels and our overall health.

6) Maintaining a steady level of hydration helps keep your body temperature stable, offsets muscle stiffness, helps regulate blood pressure, participates in the body's waste disposal system and assists in the transport of nutrients and oxygen throughout the body. Keeping a steady level of hydration eases aging and offsets a plethora of potential issues.

7) Many of the issues we attribute to aging should be blamed on the real culprit: misuse of our bodies and lack of care. There is a recurring theme found in scientific studies on aging that shows if you want to extend your life span and stay healthy, you need to maintain a regular exercise program.

8) Sleeping well at night has everything to do with your behavior during the day, your hydration, your stress, your exercise regimen (or lack thereof), what you eat, and how you feel about life – your happiness.

9) Instead of "going on a diet," take a longer, proactive approach and change the foods you eat, make smarter choices and gradually stick to the new habits you develop.

Chapter 12
STRESS – THE SILENT SABOTEUR

*"The rush and pressure of modern life are a form,
perhaps the most common form, of its innate violence.
To allow oneself to be carried away by a multitude of
conflicting concerns, to surrender to too many demands,
to commit oneself to too many projects, to want to help
everyone in everything, is to succumb to violence."*

Thomas Merton

As Merton so vividly points out, putting yourself in stress is nothing less than creating violence against your physical being – your body – and defeating that which you think you are driven to do. It wreaks havoc on your physical self. It is how we are hard-wired.

The stress response is actually a brilliant system of checks and balances which is designed to save our lives under imminent stress. The problem is that 10,000 years ago, when we were being chased by a dangerous animal, our bodies were made to go into high gear instantly. You know it: The Fight or Flight Response.

As soon as we realized that we were in danger, this is what happens to us physically:

Stress hormones are released into our body – glucagon, cortisol, and adrenaline.

The glucagon signals a reduction in insulin production so that your blood sugar (which is spiking to give you that burst of energy) cannot be tampered with.

The cortisol triggers glucose to rush into your muscles so they have the ability to react quickly and run if necessary. Your blood actually thickens. And by the way, high cortisol levels impair your brain cognition, attention span, memory, and the processing of emotions.

Adrenaline rushes into the bloodstream to help signal the organs to react: the heart to pound faster, the blood pressure to increase, the lungs to breathe quicker. With more oxygen in the blood, the nervous system gets on board and gears up for the flight which is about to take place.

All unnecessary systems and body functions cease as they are not needed in this emergency: food digestion, immune system, hair, nail and cell growth, etc.

And this is just a very small example of the hormonal influence during the first five seconds of the fear being realized. Keep in mind, these hormones don't just stop when the stress ebbs. Rather, they can stay in the bloodstream for extended periods of time, especially cortisol.

Here we are, 10,000+ years later, and our stress response system, unfortunately, has not changed all that much. But our reasons for stress have. We now know that stress and how we manage it have a direct link to how our bodies manifest disease. Ten thousand years ago our stress was sudden, imminent and over in a short period of time. Our bodies could then calm down and we could just continue doing what we were doing. The stress was acute – short term – and critical for our survival. We, obviously, still live with acute stress which still helps with our survival, but rarely is that stress life-threatening.

The same can't be said for chronic stress. Probably the most critical change that takes place when in stress is the suppression of the immune system.

Again, when that animal is chasing you, you really don't need to ward off any germs at the time, so your immune system gets suppressed. A *chronic* suppression of the immune system, and those increased cortisol levels supporting it, can result in more frequent colds, bronchitis, headaches, increased blood sugar levels, brain fog, sugar cravings, fatigue, enhanced allergies or asthma, anxiety and/or depression, slower healing of a wound, sexual impotence, chest pains, high blood pressure, migraines, heartburn, digestive issues, constipation, dry mouth, muscle cramping, irregular menses…need I go on? Then there are the outer signs that reveal that your body is being bombarded by stress: acne, dry skin, circles under the eyes, thinning hair, warts, oily scalp, sweating more, rosacea, psoriasis, eczema and lots more. Bottom line is that if your body and mind are in a constant state of stress, the potential for disease is enormous. That, obviously, needs to change.

THE MANY FACES OF STRESS

Please understand that how chronic stress manifests in my body is totally different than how it manifests in yours. We each have our more vulnerable place where stress likes to simmer. My mother, for instance, always had back issues, for as long as I could remember. It started when she actually did put her back out, picking up either my brother or myself from the bathtub when we were toddlers. That triggered a vulnerability to her back. When she got into the full swing of being a working mom (in the 60s when there were very few women who did that) her stress would build through the school year (she worked in school administration). Then, every year in June, she would "put her back out." She would end up in bed for about a week, then slowly but surely, by July, her back would be fine. Her body would stave off the trauma until the school year was over (her source of stress) and it was safe to collapse. By July, her mindset and determination would heal her back and she was good to go. Through the decades, doctors could not find anything wrong with her back and no "scars" from that initial injury.

Most people don't have such an obvious annual wakeup call. Instead, they endure the stress they live with and are oblivious to the disease simmering in their bodies, often in the form of heart disease or cancer. But more and more studies show the relationship of disease to stress, especially autoimmune disease. And, we are finally beginning to understand how interconnected our stress is to our emotions.

I firmly believe that my atrial fibrillation was my wakeup call. It actually started in my childhood, when I was about 12 years old. The doctor gave some convoluted explanation of an athletic heart, which didn't really make any sense to me, though I did participate in sports. And he only said this to me. He told my mom I was fine. What I now know after dealing with AFib for 50+ years is that when I was 12, I had a broken heart. I lived in a stressful home with two working parents who didn't particularly like each other, neither of whom had much time for their kids. My brother would stay to himself in his room and I was left alone most of the time. By the time I was 12, my self-worth was zero and my heart was broken from loneliness. My heart became my vulnerable spot.

Consider different conditions that could be correlated with your stress. Suspend your disbelief for a moment and think about how your stress and emotions might be manifesting themselves in your body:

If you have a lung issue, could it be that you are suffocating a part of you, that you are not able to be your true self or speak in your own voice?

If you are chronically constipated, aside from not being hydrated enough, could you be holding things in and not being honest with yourself or your loved ones?

If you suffer from headaches or migraines, are you too often coming from your head and not your heart, over-taxing your brain, especially with stressful thoughts?

Could your rheumatoid arthritis be tied into an inability to be flexible as a person and perhaps you are too set in your ways?

Okay, call me crazy or completely disagree with me. But I heard of a woman who suffered from throat cancer after keeping a critical lie from her husband for many years. She was not speaking her truth. I suspect this kind of thing could be happening to many of us. All I ask you to do is consider that whatever issue you may be having physically could, in fact, tie into an emotional issue. And by living with chronic stress, your chances of manifesting illness in that area are much greater.

My main point is for you to recognize that your body communicates to you in many ways. Being in "dis-ease" is just one of them. Our society dictates that doctors know how to cure us. Doctors are not taught the correlation between your body and your mind, your spirit, your emotions or your stress. So, this aspect of your health is not always available to them, and consequently, to you. I am simply suggesting that you take a look at the body part that seems to have given you trouble over the years and see if its function could possibly be related to an emotional hot button for you. It might not be. But, just for fun, think about it. And also take note of *when* it seems to speak to you – was it during times of increased stress?

WHERE DOES STRESS REALLY COME FROM?

As mentioned, there are two different kinds of stress. Acute stress, which occurs instantly when exposed to a specific trigger, and chronic stress, which starts with a specific trigger but continues over time and lingers, often for years, even decades. It is chronic stress which can give us the most trouble physically and, ironically, the stress over which we have the most control.

When you think about it, stress is created by how we react to a particular situation. Think for a few seconds of something that has happened to you that is causing you to be stressed. You realize you are stressed because you can't seem to sleep very well at night, you are snacking more than usual, you have become overly chatty with anyone who will listen or you are much quieter than usual, you tend to lose patience with everyone who does not have an immediate answer for you, you are impatient when driving, you may have one more drink than you typically do, or – the big one – you can't stop thinking about it! Emotionally, you feel frustrated or anxious or sad or angry or scared or some other emotion that is alarming for you. If I haven't hit on any behavior changes or emotions that you have experienced, I am sure that you can come up with your own. Since that incident happened, what are you doing differently, even if it is minor?

As time goes on, day after day, are the changed behaviors continuing? Do you keep having that pit in your stomach when you think about what happened? Are people beginning to notice this new you or are you pretty much able to keep it concealed?

So, here's an idea – what if all you needed to do was change how you think about the incident that happened? If you are blaming someone else for it, what if you took full responsibility? If someone else has caused this hurt, what if you forgave them? After all, no one else can control how you think – that is all yours. What if you could simply think differently about what happened? By thinking differently, you don't change what happened. But you can completely change your perspective and let go of the thinking that was stressing you out. As the title of Wayne Dyer's book, <u>Change Your Thoughts, Change Your Life,</u> suggests, by changing your thoughts you let go of the stress that was connected to the incident, and therefore you change how your body reacts to it.

In other words, you have complete control over how you react to whatever situation befalls you. The emotion derived because of your thought process will then determine the effect that the incident takes on your physiology. If your thoughts are upbeat and positive, you will create all those good-feeling hormones and feel good – your own dose of good medicine for the mind, body and spirit.

If, however, you feel the need to get angry, resentful and regretful, in time those emotions and their accompanying stress will eat away at your physicality, compounding with whatever other negativity is going on. In time, the incident could then be the catalyst, or at least a contributor, to some form of disease which will show up in due time.

THE HIDDEN FACES OF STRESS

I think it is pretty safe to say we are usually aware of when we are in stress. But I would like to present some alternative circumstances which we may not realize are causing us stress. This is just a small sampling which I hope will get you thinking of situations you have been going through over the years that you did not consider being stressful.

Past Trauma and Forgiveness

What if you had a car accident that you caused when you were 36, totaling your own car and someone else's, sending you both to the hospital with injuries, where you both slowly recovered. But did you? Have you confronted that trauma head on and absolved yourself and let it go? If not, it could be festering inside of you and you don't even know it.

Underlying stress is often from trauma that occurred at some point in your life, perhaps more than once. It doesn't have to be trauma from an incident or accident. It can be from a relationship breaking up, loss of a close friend, relative or child. You could be in a job that you love with a boss that you hate. You could be burying your true feelings and opinions from everyone to avoid confrontation. You could be going through life without really speaking your mind and no one knows that but you.

Oftentimes these integrated stressors have simply become a part of our lives. Whatever the trigger, it could have happened a long time ago, or it could still be going on. But the stress is ever-present in you, lying just beneath the surface. It might be possible to get rid of that stress through forgiveness.

You cannot change what happened and you cannot control how the other person/people behave or react, if there are others involved. You don't have to reconcile with anyone or condone what they did. You can only control your emotions and memories of what happened. The priority is to do what is right for you to finally put the matter behind you, learn from it and put it to rest. As I am sure you have heard, forgiveness is all about you, not them.

When we choose *not* to forgive, nothing good comes from that. Lack of forgiveness only fosters negative emotions in us: anger, resentment, bitterness, hate, fear, regret, disappointment. Even though we are projecting onto them, we are the ones still holding onto the emotional baggage. And that emotional baggage is what simmers as stress in our bodies day after day.

You will find a more extensive explanation of forgiveness and its importance to our emotional well-being in Chapter 14, *Mobility for Life*.

Loneliness

It is hard to imagine that in this day and age, with all the technology available to connect with people, that anyone could be lonely, but it is true. Perhaps you yearn to be in an intimate relationship and cannot seem to find that special someone. You've tried parties and blind dates and dating sites, but you can't seem to click with anyone. Your social life could be chock full and your calendar busy every day and night and yet, because you would really rather be with that one person whom you can't seem to meet, you are lonely. You may not even realize it because you are so busy. But in all the busyness, if you sense a void, it could be from feeling lonely.

Or, maybe at work, every day, you just don't seem to fit in. You love your job, but the people in the office are not really friends. You go out with them after work sometimes, but you just can't seem to make a connection.

Perhaps you have suffered the loss of a loved one and it's two years later and people don't seem to understand why you aren't "over it" yet. A piece of you is missing and, no, you aren't "over it" yet, but it doesn't mean that you aren't progressing in your healing.

Occasional loneliness happens to everybody. But chronic loneliness could be a problem. It could come from the lack of a partner, but it could also come from a lack of connection to people in general. If this goes on for months and maybe years at a time, it could affect your physiology, just like stress does. It could actually be construed as stress, though the symptoms are very different. Stress tends to speed things up. Loneliness tends to slow things down. However, the toll it takes on the body is about the same.

The key to dealing with loneliness is to first recognize that you are, in fact, lonely. Nothing to be ashamed of. But now you have a foundation on which to grow. The most important way to deal with loneliness is to realize that you are your own best partner. You are your own best friend. To melt loneliness away, you need to fall in love with yourself. And, by falling in love with yourself, you will never be lonely again.

That doesn't mean that you want to be alone. It means that you want to complete yourself first, then add to your life people who will help you feel fuller and who will help you grow and thrive.

To help you fall in love with yourself, you may want to hire a professional therapist. Also, there are books and programs online that can help you with self-compassion and self-love. The important thing is to be honest with yourself about your personality and who you are as a person. Be kind. And always be able to laugh at yourself. I tend to laugh at myself at least once a day. Sometimes I am pretty funny!!

Perfectionism

There are many reasons why one evolves into a perfectionist. It can be from our childhood (seems like everything is, somehow) or our adulthood, but most perfectionists simply want to be in control. In most cases, it's not a want, but a need. Regardless of how this started, if you recognize that you have perfectionist tendencies, it would behoove you to pay attention and try to "let it go."

Perfectionism comes in different levels. Some people are so obsessed that if they walk into a chaotic room, it is very difficult for them to feel comfortable. Others are like Felix Unger in *The Odd Couple* and require everything in their environment to be neat and in its place. Some can work on something for hours to get it just right. Others can take days or more. The hard part with being a perfectionist is that you are not aware of the underlying toll it is taking on your nervous system and the rest of your body.

If you need things to always be a certain way, it is painful when they aren't. And if you are not in a position to fix the situation, your body is churning.

If this is you, you need to first recognize that letting perfectionism go is not an easy task. After that, you may want to figure out whom else this trait of yours is affecting. Those behaviors that affect others would be the first to work on. (You may want to wait until you finish Chapter 13, *Your Fiscal Physical Retirement Plan*, and use the weaning chart I offer there. Substitute behaviors for the food items and you can create your own calendar of behavior modification.)

Perfectionism can also serve you. The key is knowing when it is serving you versus when it is interfering. But to help with the stress it creates, it is very important that you recognize it. That way you can help yourself relax and let some things go. And by letting up on some of that self-made pressure you can reduce the stress it is creating.

Vanity

Does it sometimes take you hours to get ready to go out? Do you change outfits a half a dozen times to find just the right one? Does putting on makeup take a half an hour or more? And your hair another half-hour or more? Believe me, there is no judgment here. I just have never known how to spend that much time getting ready. Yet for some, it can be a daily occurrence.

I by no means am suggesting that this is a bad thing. What I am suggesting is to ask yourself if you are having a good time doing it. If you enjoy taking that amount of time getting ready and feel fabulous when you walk out the door, then keep it up! It not only serves your ego, but enhances your nervous system and the overall "feeling good" part of your physiology. If, however, you are continuously frustrated by the process and indecisive about each step you go through, then you are creating stress in your body each morning, and over time it will take its toll. I do encourage you to curb the behavior, if necessary, to help alleviate the stress it may be causing.

Being the Center of Attention

If you are this person, you probably don't even know it. But everybody else does. Psychology 101 would say it stems from insecurity felt in childhood and never getting enough attention. It could manifest as anything from comedic behavior to non-stop talking. The important thing to know is that if you are not getting the attention you need, you will have stress in your body.

Again, I would call on professional help so that you will be able to get to the root of this issue. When your needs are not being fulfilled, it creates stress. Since needing attention is pretty much a full time trait, I would guess that your body is in a state of chronic stress. Therefore, this trait is aging you too quickly and potentially creating the foundation for an upcoming disease.

Please understand that I am not a psychologist, therapist or licensed clinical social worker. In all cases of dealing with psychological issues, I encourage you to seek professional help. But, if you do not choose that route, I hope that some of these suggestions are helpful in learning more about yourself. They are not the complete solution, of course, but as a personal trainer for over 20 years, I have found these suggestions beneficial in alleviating chronic stress.

One fun and healthy thing to do is to study your traits to determine their origin in your childhood. Sometimes we are sitting on our own answers. I mentioned my loneliness as a child; I recognized the basis for it and then changed my behavior to honor it.

Perfectionism is another trait I have dealt with. Believe me, I am much better than I used to be. At least whatever perfectionism I deal with now doesn't really impose on anyone but me. I got my perfectionism from my dad and whenever I see myself going that way, I laugh and say, "Thanks, Dad!! This is all your fault!"

You are who you are. You are a magnificent human being here to live your journey and help and support others along the way. When you notice a personality trait that might be imposing on the flow of your everyday life, stop and take a look at it. If it's not hurting anyone else and it doesn't bother you *and* it is not causing you stress, then embrace it and love it as a part of who you are.

ENERGY – STRESS' SECRET RESOURCE

Although what has been presented makes stress seem like a really bad thing except in emergency situations, I would also like to suggest to you that the stress you experience may be turned to your advantage.

Athletes, for instance, are often trained to refocus the stress they feel before a game or competition. If they sense nervousness or anxiety, they recognize it for what it is and choose to view it as additional energy for their body to use to improve their performance.

There was a study done with a small group of students. They were given instructions to "reinterpret physical stress symptoms as energy." They scored higher and reported less emotional exhaustion before taking a stressful exam.[69]

I have done quite a bit of public speaking in my career. No matter how comfortable I was with the topic or venue or length of the speech I was about to give, I got butterflies in my stomach. Quite frankly, I don't know anyone who is about to go on stage that doesn't get a hint of them. At one event, I was chatting with a woman who was about to go on right ahead of me. She was someone I admired and far more experienced than I. She flat out asked if I were nervous – did I have butterflies? No shame here, I said that I did. And right before she walked on stage, she turned to me and said, "embrace them!"

---

[69] *IDEA Fitness Journal,* February 2017

I have never forgotten that and never will. I took her sage advice and now don't really get many butterflies anymore, but when I do, I embrace them and the stress goes away!

Thinking differently and believing what you are thinking are the real secrets to realigning stress into a more positive energy for your health and your body. Next time you are heading into what you know will be a difficult scenario, try to use that stress energy by applying it toward a positive outcome. See how much calmer and more control you feel throughout the experience. Stress doesn't have to be a bad thing.

As a matter of fact, stress can be a good thing when it shows up in a desperate situation. I remember once being with a friend in her backyard where she had a pool. The kids were having a great time and we were being good moms, watching them constantly. All of a sudden, my baby girl of nine months, who had been happily sitting in a seated inflatable ring, sank to the bottom of the pool. I leapt up, took two giant steps and jumped in. She was not in the deep end, so I bent over, picked her up and pulled her up into the air. I had a huge smile on my face and said "Wow, sweetie!! Wasn't that fun?" She blinked the water away from her eyes and had a completely startled look on her face. Fortunately, because I had this big grin on my face, she started to giggle. In the meantime, my entire body was on high stress alert and stayed that way, slowly ebbing as minutes ticked by. Needless to say, I was incredibly grateful that I went into my acute stress mode without any conscious thinking at all. It was a built-in, full-tilt stress reaction.

Our bodies are incredibly brilliant, manipulating our systems to work together to save us from the man-eating beast of 10,000 years ago, or from an annoying boss who is always on our case. This helps us cope and even survive. But when stress extends its reach within our body, it can create debilitating and life-threatening diseases if left unchecked. It is important to recognize its impact on our health and physicality. Though it can take decades to manifest into something debilitating, it is wise to pay attention along the way so that you can stay in front of it and have it work for your health and not against it. And if you are carrying some old stress around, perhaps it is time to let it go.

Several strategies for letting go of stress are explored throughout this book and suggested here: meditation, mindfulness, breathing, exercise, walking, being in nature, positive mental imaging, taking breaks, music, venting to someone, therapy, having a spiritual practice, redirecting how you think, better diet, tensing then releasing your entire body ... and the list goes on and on. Find out what will work for you and what you will stick to. This is a life-long commitment because there will always be stress in your life. It is how you manage it that will determine its impact on you.

CHAPTER 12 RECAP

1) The stress response is actually a brilliant system of checks and balances designed to save our lives under imminent stress. Back in the caveman days, to save us from a dangerous beast, our Fight or Flight Response was triggered. Today, that same response exists, but turning it off has become a problem.

2) Nowadays, the stress that was a dangerous animal could be a boss or a husband or a parent. Our stress today is typically chronic and not short-lived.

3) If your body and mind are in a constant state of stress, the potential for disease is enormous.

4) Whatever physical issue you may be having could tie into an emotional issue. And by living with chronic stress, your chances of manifesting illness in that area are much greater.

5) Your body communicates to you in many ways. Being in dis-ease is just one of them.

6) Some sample sources of stress include past traumas, inability to forgive, loneliness, perfectionism, vanity, or needing to be the center of attention.

7) Next time you are heading into what you know will be a difficult scenario, use your imagination to turn that stress energy into a positive outcome for you.

8) Thinking differently – and believing what you are thinking – are the real secrets to realigning stress into a more positive energy for your health and your body.

9) Though some stressful scenarios can take decades to manifest into something debilitating, it is wise to pay attention along the way so that you can stay in front of it and have it work for your health and not against it. And if you are carrying some old stress around, perhaps it is time to let it go.

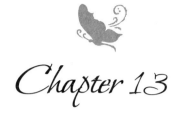

Chapter 13

YOUR ~~FISCAL~~ PHYSICAL RETIREMENT PLAN

"All you need is the plan, the road map, and the courage to press on to your destination."

Earl Nightingale

Why is it that when people try to determine how much money they will need to retire, they do not consider what their physical condition will need to be in order to ensure that all their retirement savings isn't spent on their failing health? After all, when you think about it, if you don't have your health when you retire, what good is your nest egg if you have to use it to pay for your poor health? I have other ideas for my retirement savings!!

A grim result from a study by the Department of Medicine, Cambridge Hospital at Harvard Medical School: "Using a conservative definition, 62.1% of all bankruptcies in 2007 were medical; 92% of these medical debtors had medical debts over $5,000, or 10% of pretax family income. The rest met criteria for medical bankruptcy because they had lost significant income due to illness or mortgaged a home to pay medical bills. Most medical debtors were well-educated, owned homes, and had middle-class occupations. Three quarters had health insurance."[70]

> *Planning for retirement is not only about finances. It's about your physicality, too!*

When thinking of retirement, every one of us needs to give equal consideration to our health *and* to our finances.

I believe we are more aware of this now than ever before. We are bombarded with messages suggesting a healthier lifestyle. Unfortunately, awareness does not necessarily change behavior.

The fitness industry is doing everything in its power to present a plethora of ways to offset the inevitability of aging, but in many cases the options are too difficult, unavailable or uninspiring. The growing availability of organic food in the marketplace, the warnings of GMOs in our food, and the rise in farmers' market products are proof positive that people are more aware of what they are eating and that diet plays a significant role in their health. The enrollment rate at gyms and health clubs is skyrocketing by those over age forty-five, because they know it is best to start exercising earlier rather than later. "The U.S. has more gyms – over 32,270 – than it has McDonald's, Dunkin' Donuts and Taco Bells combined."[71]

So why aren't the health statistics better than they are? Why do they continue to show results of declining health, not improvements?

Why are more people being diagnosed with life debilitating diseases, and at a younger age?

Why is the obesity rate still climbing?

I believe many people are trying. But they are failing. And they try again and fail again. It then becomes a cycle of frustration and disappointment.

---

[70] nih.org (National Institutes of Health), US National Library of Medicine, "Medical Bankruptcy in the United States 2007: Results of a National Study"
[71] *AARP Bulletin*, May 2022

In the weight loss category alone, it is reported that 65% of people who lose weight gain it back, and often they gain back more.[72]

We deserve to retire both fiscally *and* physically fit.

WHAT IF THERE WERE A PLAN?

A plan that was progressive in nature but didn't require taking huge steps one at a time from the start? What if there were a check-and-balance system so that you are always moving towards the ultimate goal? What if the plan were designed to inspire and encourage you, with a realistic approach? What if the plan were unique to you: customized for your specific dreams and desires, your specific capabilities and your specific dietary needs?

And, what if you had twenty years to complete the plan?

WHY TWENTY YEARS?

Looking back, twenty years seems like either forever ago or it can seem like ten minutes ago!

When I think of twenty years ago, I think of where I was living, who I was living with, what job I had, where my children were, friends, what I was doing – all sorts of things. As I reflect, I look at how much was accomplished and the experiences I lived through. As I think of the *next* twenty years, I have visions of dreams yet to be lived! Twenty years from now, as I write this, I will be over 90. There is a whole lot of life to be lived between now and then!

At this stage of your life, you know how quickly twenty years fly by.

---

[72] livestrong.com, "The Percentage of People Who Regain Weight After Rapid Weight Loss and the Risks of Doing So"

In all my training and educating throughout the years spent in this industry, I have never heard a single suggestion that this transition was going to take a long time, that it could take up to twenty years to *completely change a lifestyle*. In fact, we see the exact opposite in both the diet and fitness worlds. People want a quick fix, so the diet and fitness gurus give it to them! They do this in the form of exercise plans that only take ten minutes of your day and promise you will achieve extreme body reform! Then there are the diet programs where you can lose 10 pounds in two weeks! So, twenty years simply seems like it is way too long a period of time to give you the results you want *now*.

But let me ask you. How long did it take for you to get where you are today? Could it be something close to or maybe even more than twenty years? Here I am 25 years later, and my 20-year plan has worked!

Some changes came easily, but most took some time – a lot of time. Lifestyle habits and behaviors are hard to change, no matter how good they are for you. My baby girl is now 30 years old and I am proud to say there is not one physical activity she can dream up at which I cannot match her, and sometimes beat her!! And she is pretty fit! Admittedly, throughout the twenty-plus years of making those changes, there were a few restarts. I imagine it might be the same for you. And that is okay. As long as you do what I did – I kept my "eye on the prize" and kept progressing in the right direction. It took perseverance! It took commitment! It took persistence! And giving myself twenty years turns out to have been more realistic than I knew at the time.

How long it will take YOU *is entirely up to you*. I have had clients do it all in less than a year, only to relapse time and time again. The most successful clients (those who have changed their behavior and stuck with it over time) took, on average, 3-5 years to really solidify all behaviors into their new lifestyle. The 20-year plan was right for me simply because that is how long it took me!! And I don't want you to give up if that is how long it takes you.

YOUR ~~FISCAL~~ PHYSICAL RETIREMENT PLAN

The Hare and the Tortoise

A Hare was making fun of the Tortoise one day for being so slow. "Do you ever get anywhere?" he asked with a mocking laugh?

"Yes," replied the Tortoise, "and I get there sooner than you think. I'll run you a race and prove it."

The Hare was much amused at the idea of running a race with the Tortoise, but for the fun of the thing he agreed.

So the Fox, who had consented to act as judge, marked the distance and started the runners off.

The Hare was soon far out of sight, and to make the Tortoise feel very deeply how ridiculous it was for him to try a race with a Hare, he lay down beside the course to take a nap until the tortoise should catch up.

The Tortoise, meanwhile, kept going slowly but steadily, and, after a time, passed the place where the Hare was sleeping.

But the Hare slept on very peacefully; and when at last he did wake up, the Tortoise was near the goal.

The Hare ran his swiftest, but he could not overtake the Tortoise in time.[73]

The moral of this story is...
Slow and steady wins the race.

The moral of your 20-year plan is...
Long-term commitment and perseverance will lead you to your dreams and desires.

THE BIGGEST HURDLE: "I-DON'T-CARE-ITIS"

According to Dr. Steven Aldana, "… 'I-don't-care-itis' is a common condition in which an individual has no interest in adopting a healthy lifestyle."[74] I am not sure if people have no interest, but they certainly do not make successful efforts to change their patterns in order to assure a healthier lifestyle and a healthier body. You may feel that this is an unfair statement. I wish it were. "70% of annual deaths in the U.S. are caused

---

[73] loc.gov (Library of Congress), read.gov/aesop
[74] <u>The Culprit and the Cure</u>, Steven G. Aldana, PhD, Chapter 3

by chronic diseases; these *preventable* diseases are also the leading cause of disability…6 in 10 adults have a chronic disease."[75]

If so many diseases are preventable, why are so many people sick? Is Dr. Aldana right? Do people really have no interest and do not care? Has our society become too spoiled to do the work necessary to succeed in healthy living? Has the medical industry gotten us too conditioned to simply take a pill to fix ourselves?

My explanation is a bit more all-encompassing. Simply put: We are a reactionary society. We are not a proactive one. It is very difficult for us to try to prevent something from happening. It is more likely that we will wait for the disaster then try to fix it once it hits.

As an example, if we were more proactive, man's participation in climate change would not exist because we would have prevented it when the potential was first hypothesized back in 1896. Even back then, it was suggested that carbon dioxide emissions from the burning of fossil fuels (coal) would eventually raise the earth's temperature. We had another opportunity to be proactive in the 1930s with warnings that the "greenhouse effect" was coming, raising the earth's temperature. Then again, in the '50s and '60s when calculations became more sophisticated and the numbers were beginning to show that there was, in fact, something happening, we could have been more proactive then. Finally, we reached the 1970s and found ourselves paying a bit more attention to our environment, accepting that the theories are more plausible. [76] Unfortunately, politics and money took over and the rest, as they say, is history.

Even with something this imminent in our future, we are not able to change our behavior. As the weather gets worse and the coastlines get smaller, our behavior may change from reactive to proactive, but right now, it seems we only react to whatever actually hits us personally.

---

[75] drhyman.com, "How Disease Impacts the Economy," May 9, 2019
[76] *Scientific American,* "The Discovery of Global Warming," August 17, 2012

The same is true of our health. We know that cakes and cookies and sodas and red meat and fried foods are not healthy for us, yet we continue to eat them. Some of us eat this way daily! There just seems to be little or no thought of our own future health. You might not know how a hamburger and fries today are going to impact your life at age 85. The simple answer is, accumulatively. We now know that children as young as age twelve are shown to have fatty deposits in their blood systems due to improper diets. *At age 12!* Let that accumulate over another 20-40 years and boom! A heart attack by age 50, or even younger! I just heard from a friend of mine that she lost a friend from a heart attack at 48! Left behind a wife and three children. That certainly wasn't the plan for that family.

However, if you have not, to date, been successful in creating a workable plan for your healthy physical future, rest assured you can start one now! The remainder of this chapter is dedicated to teaching you the various ways to do it and the parts of your lifestyle on which to focus.

CHANGING YOUR FOOD HABITS

What are your food habits and how do you change these lifelong eating behaviors?

It is important to respect the amount of time our food journey has taken to bring us to where we are now. Recognizing that these changes did not happen overnight helps to relieve the pressure we may feel to hurry up and change everything immediately. By taking away the pressure for immediate results, you allow yourself to adjust and move forward with successes in baby steps – smaller stages and phases. You also remove the difficulty of making too many changes all at the same time, which I believe is what causes failure for many. And if you simply stop eating junk food all at once, depending on how much of your diet consists of these foods, you will most likely go into a form of detox and feel exhausted, nauseous and quite ill for a good week or more. Another good reason for you to take it one step at a time.

Take note, it probably will not take you 20 years to make all the changes you want to make, but in the big picture, 20 years is a good mindset to start with. Then, when you fulfill your dreams in 5 years, you will be oh-so-very proud! The journey starts with food. That in itself is a long road of discovery.

One of the critical and most difficult things for me to give up was sugar. I am pretty sure we all have the same challenge – we are a nation of people who love our sweets! To repeat the statistics in Chapter 9, *You Are What You Eat*, the U.S. Department of Agriculture states that the average person consumes 156 pounds of sugar each year! That is almost 1 cup of sugar each day per person! That figure is astounding. But remember all the foods that contain sugar - keeping in mind that simple carbohydrates are processed as sugar in our bodies, so it is not just the sweet stuff.

I loved all things meant to be sweet - cookies, cake, pie, ice cream – anything called dessert! For most of my life I tried desperately to avoid these delicious temptations. I was so addicted to sugar, that I often couldn't drive by a specific store without making a pit-stop to get a specific "treat." For me, the start of success meant I had to change my route! I had to stop driving by that store. It was hard! I am not going to lie – there were times I thought it would be okay just once… but as a month passed, then two, I was good. I could now drive past that store without stopping, even though the desire was still there.

This is just one example of a change I had to make. Again, the point I want to emphasize is that there are a lot of changes you will be making. The list is very extensive and they all are part of individual habits you have developed over the years and now need to change. If you Google "Books on Changing Habits," there are thousands of answers for you. Each author has his or her own theories about why it takes time to change a habit. But typically, although some say 21 days and others say 90 days and still others say 6 months, truth be told, it will take as long as it takes FOR YOU! Knowing yourself better than anybody, you may want to create your own timeframes and develop your own schedule as time goes on. You will be able to realize through your own determination how long changing your behavior will take with each step.

And, even then, there can be regressions – our will and determination can be overtaken by our desire – the memory of that moment of pleasure on the tongue. Behavior change is hard and regressions happen, but each time I "cheated" it was a little less damaging than the previous time – that is a victory you have to accept!

I am sure sugar elimination is going to be a part of your own personal habit change. It is a much bigger category than most are aware of, and it truly is the most difficult shift to make in your eating habits. The following will help you understand why this habit is so hard to overcome.

Sugar has been found to be 8 times more addictive than cocaine! And even more discouraging is that sugar is not found in just desserts and sweets, but also in cereals, breads, crackers, pastas, chips – and more! It would be safe to say that almost all processed foods are contributing to your sugar intake. As explained in Chapter 9, flour breaks down into simple carbohydrates. The human body identifies this as sugar and processes it in the same way it does table sugar.

Dairy and gluten are two other food groups that many people give up, for the same reasons as giving up sugar. These food groups create inflammation in most people. And as we have discussed, inflammation creates building blocks for everything from cancer to Alzheimer's. The same goes for meat – it, too, creates inflammation in your body. If your choice is to slowly, but surely, eliminate these sorts of foods from your life, you may better understand why it can take so many years to do it.

I will admit, my friends and family call me an extremist and I have to agree. But this is my body and this is my choice for taking care of my future health. It has worked exceptionally well for me in that I simply don't get sick. Typical aging symptoms that start to creep in by the time you are 70 are arthritis or achy joints, hay fever or pollen allergies, a weaker immune system, osteopenia or osteoporosis – weaker bones, shrunken height…. People typically lose an inch by now. They gain weight, or a pot belly. As of now, none of these is happening to me. In fact, I had osteopenia for years and my last bone density test showed that the trend is reversing!

As mentioned before, I have also suffered from atrial fibrillation (heart palpitations and rapid heartbeat or very slow sporadic beats) since I was a child – 12 years old. It has been dormant for most of my life, but it came back with a vengeance several years ago. It was only when I had my food sensitivity blood test and stopped eating the foods that were inflammatory to my system that episodes became few and far between, if at all. I also began to meditate on a regular basis which I know also contributed to the lessening of episodes. As previously discussed, the direct connection between the heart and the mind have shown up for me before. As soon as I got my stress under control, and was "perfect" with my diet, I got my AFib under control. (I am by no means recommending that you handle AFib yourself. You need to discuss it with your doctor and do what is right for you. I am only telling you this because it demonstrates how better decisions and habit changes can benefit you and your future health.) As of this writing, AFib episodes are very rare and of a very short duration. Before that it was 24/7 (with occasional 1-2 day reprieves) for the last 6 years!

THE BOTTOM LINE

The bottom line for optimal health is knowing that most disease is caused by inflammation, and most inflammation is caused by stress, toxins and food. Because food choices and how we oversee our stress are completely under our control, we can change, manage, and eliminate inflammation and most toxins. (Non-food toxins can be handled with another method, which I discuss later in this chapter.)

Foods slowly eliminated over time, based on what is right and not right *for you*, can help to eliminate chronic inflammation. This strengthens your immune system and allows your body to maintain a higher level of homeostasis (balance) which is all your body wants and continuously strives to maintain. The more support we give to our bodies to be in homeostasis, the healthier we are.

I have chosen to eat a very restrictive diet that has taken me more than twenty years to develop and adapt to. It is one of the steps I have taken to control my own aging. Your road may be different and that is okay. But you *do* need to find the healthiest food plan that is customized and works best for you. Remember, your food plan is for YOUR body. Depending on whatever issues you may currently be living with that are affected by diet (such as diabetes) make sure you discuss your plans with your doctor.

DESIGNING YOUR FOOD PLAN

The most successful way to move forward in designing your food plan is with baby steps -- by taking just one habit/behavior at a time and breaking it down to its smallest component. Success is the goal, not constantly retreating, cheating or quitting. Every change you make needs a simple methodology you can follow easily so that you can't help but succeed. Listen to yourself as you walk through this plan – if you sense you will fail, make it easier! Break the pieces of change down even further. One baby step at a time.

Five Steps to Creating Your Food Plan

This is the start of your journey. It might seem like an inordinate amount of work, but it is important. When you are moving forward after this, you will thank yourself for going through this process.

To begin, please do the following exercise which will take you quite a few minutes to complete. Sit with it and really think through every single thing you eat that you know you shouldn't – even if you don't eat it very often, but it is something you know is unhealthy for you.

Step 1: Start by making a list of ALL the foods you like to eat that you know are not the best choices. When in doubt, add them to the list – most likely your intuition is letting you know what you don't want to admit.

Step 2: Rank each food on a scale of 1 to 10. 10 is the most difficult to quit and 1 is the easiest to quit. If your list is really not that long – like less than 25 things, then do a scale of 1 – 5. (To date, I have never had a client with fewer than 25 foods!)

Step 3: Group the various foods together by their assigned number. Put all the foods that are ranked number 1 together in one group and do the same for all numbers 1-10.

Step 4: Within each of your grouped lists, 1-10, prioritize the foods in each group, listing the easiest ones to give up at the top and the hardest ones to give up down at the bottom.

Congratulate yourself for a job well done! This was a lot of work, but I think you can already see the benefits of doing this and how important it is to your success. How are you feeling looking at your lists? Are you scared about how many foods are on your list? Are you worried you cannot eliminate all of these? Are you sad because you are really going to miss some of them?

Step 5: Now you are going to establish the time frame it will take you on your personal journey to quit these foods one at a time. Please let me reassure you. As you begin this journey and your body starts responding, you will be amazed that some of the foods you thought you could not live without you actually can live without – and others you won't miss at all! You will be pleasantly surprised to discover that some of the foods can still be a choice, just on a more limited basis.

You are giving your body a healthy cleansing so that should you choose to add that food back into your diet again, you will be able to easily see how your body handles it, and whether it is a good or a bad food choice for you. This is done by doing a one-bite- or one-serving-at-a-time test. Make sure it is at least one month since you have had that particular food. When you choose to reintroduce a food, try to take just one bite, or have just one single serving of that food. Wait a few hours, even a day, and your body should let you know how it handles this particular food.

Pay close attention to any discomfort this food brings to your body. It will be clear that this food is just not worth eating again. That's when you know you are truly on the side of a healthy future, making the best choices for your body. Congratulations again!

And while this may seem obvious, I must point out that in order for your body to be truly clean from a particular food, you need to be cleansed of that *entire* food type. Let's say you like both chocolate ice cream and black raspberry ice cream. You need to stop eating *all* ice cream, not just one or the other. In other words, just because you stopped eating chocolate ice cream for two months doesn't mean that you can keep eating black raspberry ice cream. It is the ice cream creating the discomfort, not the flavoring of the ice cream.

The chart below shows you a sample of how to set up Steps 1–5. As admitted, this is laborious, so perhaps take several days or weeks to finish. When you have it all set up with realistic time frames, all you then have to do is follow the plan. I used anywhere from 1 to 4 weeks to give up a particular item of food. You may need a shorter period of time or a longer one. That is entirely up to you. You are setting yourself up to succeed so give yourself enough time to successfully eliminate each food on the list.

SAMPLE: My Food Elimination Plan

Food Item	Level of Difficulty to Give Up (1=Easiest to Give Up)
Sugars	
Cheesecake	5
Candy: Chocolate	10
All Other Kinds of Candy	7
Ice Cream: Vanilla	10
Moose Tracks	6
Mint Chocolate Chip	8
Chocolate Chip	7
Black Raspberry	8
All Other Flavors of Ice Cream	5
Cookies: Oatmeal	4
Chocolate Chip	8
Molasses	7
All Other Kinds of Cookies	5
Protein Bars -	3
(check their sugar count: 4g = 1 tsp)	
Pie	3
Cake	3
Doughnuts	2
Brownies	5
Commercialized*	1
Simple Carbohydrates	
Potato Chips: Regular	2
Kettle Cooked	5
Stone Wheat Crackers	6
Corn Chips	1
Tortilla Chips	8
Rice Crackers	9
Commercialized*	1
Pita Chips	7
Popcorn	2
Bread - Not sprouted wheat	10
Cereal	6
Pasta	10

*By commercialized, I mean the pre-packaged, pre-labeled brands you see advertised. They usually have a long list of ingredients, half of which you don't understand, and tons of preservatives so they last for weeks. I don't want to name the brands here, but I am sure you know what foods I am referring to.

YOUR ~~FISCAL~~ PHYSICAL RETIREMENT PLAN

Sample – My Food Elimination Schedule

Food in Order of Elimination	Time it Will Take	Calendar
Commercialized* Sugars	1 Week	Jan 1 – 7
Commercialized* Carbs	1 Week	Jan 8 – 14
Corn Chips	1 Week	Jan 15 – 21
Popcorn	1 Week	Jan 22 – 28
Doughnuts	1 Week	Jan 29 – Feb 4
Potato Chips: Regular	1 Week	Feb 5 – 11
Pie	1 Week	Feb 12 – 18
Cake	1 Week	Feb 19 – 25
Protein Bars	1 Week	Feb 26 – Mar 4
Oatmeal Cookies	1 Week	Mar 5 – 11
Cheesecake	1 Week	Mar 12 – 18
Brownies	1 Week	Mar 19 – 25
Potato Chips: Kettle Cooked	1 Week	Mar 26 – Apr 1
Cookies: All Other Kinds	2 Weeks	Apr 2 – 15
Ice Cream: All Other Flavors	2 Weeks	Apr 16 – 29
Stone Wheat Crackers	2 Weeks	Apr 30 – May 13
Ice Cream: Moose Tracks	1 Week	May 14 - 20
Cereal	2 Weeks	May 21 – June 3
Cookies: Molasses	1 Week	June 4 – 10
Pita Chips	1 Week	June 11 – 17
Ice Cream: Chocolate Chip	2 Weeks	June 18 – July 1
Candy: All Other Kinds	3 Weeks	July 2 – 22
Ice Cream: Black Raspberry	2 Weeks	July 23 – Aug 5
Tortilla Chips	2 Weeks	Aug 6 – Aug 19
Cookies: Chocolate Chip	2 Weeks	Aug 20 – Sep 2
Rice Crackers	2 Weeks	Sep 3 – Sep16
Ice Cream: Mint Choc. Chip	3 Weeks	Sep 17 – Oct
Pasta	4 Weeks	Oct 8 – Nov 4
Ice Cream: Vanilla	4 Weeks	Nov 5 – Dec 2
Bread	4 Weeks	Dec 3 – 30
Candy: Chocolate	4 Weeks	Dec 31 – Jan 27
Candy: Dark Chocolate	Still consume - little to no sugar!	

Tips for Elimination Success

Within each time period, it is recommended that you wean off the food versus going cold turkey. If you know you will do better with the cold turkey approach, please do what works for you. In my experience working with clients on this, most found success in weaning off. For me it took four weeks to eliminate milk chocolate and all the other yummy ways chocolate comes (except dark, 80%). I reduced my consumption from four pieces a day down to none and it was easier to do this by lowering my consumption week by week.

Tip 1: You Don't Have to Do This Alone

By now, you are probably thinking, I'm never going to do all that!

I totally understand the dilemma! I suggest that maybe you find someone to do this with. Call each other your accountability partner. Maybe you need to hire a coach who will be there to congratulate your successes! And, if you really find that you just aren't getting it done, perhaps you want to attend one of my F.I.T. Workshops (Fitness Inspiration Transformation) and do it there!

Tip 2: Food Sensitivity Testing

If you chose to take the Food Sensitivity Test, then you should absolutely start with those foods identified as high sensitivity! The remaining foods that you know you *should* avoid can be delayed until you get those high sensitivity foods out of your system.

Again, this process can take years and truly – that is OKAY! You can choose from the very start to spread it out that way.

Tip 3: Food Categorization

Let's say you make a decision to stop eating all fried foods, but you know that is a huge challenge. So, start by cutting back the number of times you eat the first fried food on your list in a month, then the second food, etc. Let's say you want to give up French fries and chicken nuggets. If you now have fries three times per week, start by cutting back to two times per week for a month, then once per week for a month, then once every 2 weeks, then once per month, until they are history. Then start with the chicken until you have it once per month. Before you know it, you have eliminated all fried foods! And believe me, your body will let you know it is *not happy* if you try to eat it again!

Tip 4: Listen to your Body

Make sure you listen to your body along the way. Your body will absolutely let you know what it likes! Say you have given up a certain food, and it has been a long, long time, but you decide to try it again, for whatever reason. Your body will let you know if it agrees with it or not!

I found this with fried clams. My daughter was a cheerleader for three years in high school and I would go to her football games in the fall, stopping at the "BEST fried clams in the state" on the way. By the time she was in her senior year, I had almost weaned off of them, but I had to go one last time. I couldn't even finish the order. Very quickly my stomach was letting me know that this was not something I should finish. No more fried foods for me!!

Fried foods, dairy and sugar tend to have the loudest and most obvious reaction from your body when you try them after elimination. The best thing you can choose to do for your optimal future health is to pay attention to the reaction, respect it, thank your body for it and then say goodbye to that food…. *forever!*

FOREVER??!!

How about just occasionally?

My question back to you, then, would be, why? How could that short, very temporary tasting of that food be worth the difficulty that your body has reacting to it, digesting it, processing the digestion and then working hard because of the inflammation that food produces?

Your body is speaking to you the only way it knows how. Why would you ignore its cries? Your body is trying desperately to communicate with you the only way it can to help you avoid the food that is doing harm to your body. How loud does it have to scream before you pay attention?

But, as always, it is your choice.

YOUR PHYSICAL RETIREMENT PLAN FOR HYDRATION

Will it take you 20 years to change your hydration habits? Probably not.

Hydration, however, is critical to health success and most likely you are not getting enough water and fluid in your system. It might also be very possible that some of the drinks you are ingesting are not healthy and should be eliminated. You can be strategic and create a plan for your hydration intake once you have evaluated and know what is good and what is bad.

Let's take a look at what you are drinking.

If you are drinking any kind of soda – diet, no caffeine, whatever it is – in the long run, you will need to give that up! I stand firm when I say there is not one healthy soda or pop on the market, no matter what the advertising says (remember, ads are for selling!)

Check the label. Typically, there is a dramatic amount of sugar, usually from high fructose corn syrup or beet sugar which, unless organic, are GMO food products. There are also dyes and preservatives, which are foreign synthetic food products and not real food, so it would naturally create inflammation and a disturbance in your system while your body tries to figure out what to do with them. Many sodas contain phosphoric acid which draws calcium out of your bones which can lead to osteoporosis.

If soda is your thing, create your plan to wean off of it! For this particular beverage, you might choose to start by creating an Elimination Chart similar to the one created for your food. Because this is a sugar drink, it is addictive and can be a rough journey, but the benefits are absolutely 100% worth it. If you are drinking the diet variety of soda, the artificial sweeteners used are proven carcinogens, known for decades. This, too, will need to be gradually eliminated. I have friends who have had a cola habit for at least 20 years. Some even switched to the diet variety. Unfortunately, they are now suffering from a plethora of health problems, including severe osteoporosis, heart health issues and diabetes.

If you need a replacement beverage, this might be a great time to infuse your own water! Try adding orange slices, cucumbers, mint – together or alone. If this is not "enough," there are many seltzers with or without flavoring. Or try plain seltzer and squeeze your own fresh lemon or lime juice into it. Try to go light on carbonated beverages. All carbonated beverages can potentially wreak havoc in your digestive system, so you may want to cut back on all that carbonation anyway. And, if you are still craving the sweet, try adding a smidge of stevia, organic and raw, of course!

Caffeinated beverages such as coffee and tea should, as a rule, also be limited. For coffee, the general recommendation is to drink a maximum of two cups per day. The reason is the caffeine, as well as the highly acidic nature of coffee. In very large doses, it can damage the liver. Caffeine, like nicotine, sugar and alcohol, is a legal addictive substance. If you are drinking caffeinated beverages for the kick, buzz or high they give you, then weaning off of them will take some focus and patience. I am sure you are aware that too much caffeine cannot be good for the body – artificially maintaining a high energy level is just not a good thing for the body to endure. Therefore, cutting back coffee intake to 2 cups a day is the best thing you can do. Better yet, start drinking decaf if it is really the coffee you love versus the caffeine!

For caffeine elimination or reduction, I strongly suggest you withdraw slowly. You might want to do a Food Elimination Plan for these if you are a heavy consumer. By doing a slow elimination you reduce the chance of caffeine withdrawal symptoms, which are not fun. Some report the shakes, headaches, energy loss and more. You may want to start measuring how much you actually drink each day. Then literally remove one ounce at a time – maybe one ounce per week. If you drink four cups of coffee per day, the cups are most likely mugs which are about 12 ounces each. So that is 48 ounces of coffee per day. By removing one ounce of coffee per week, before the year is up, you will be caffeine free. A much easier process for your body and your caffeine addiction!

The Gold Standard for Hydration

In maintaining homeostasis, the best way to hydrate is with good old H2O!

I suggest drinking at least half of your daily hydration in water. Liquids, other than water, tend to go through the digestion process, hydrating in and around the cells, keeping the overall body hydrated as well. The *I. A.M. H.E.R.E.* chapter's section on hydration can tell you how much is enough to drink as well as other important tips about hydration.

For creating your plan to get that much fluid in your body, here is something to consider. If you rise at 6:00am and go to bed by 10:00pm, you really want all that water drunk by 6:00pm so you are not having to get up in the middle of the night. Use the suggestions in *I. A.M. H.E.R.E.* to best guide your intake.

It is also very wise to drink 8-12 ounces of water first thing in the morning. It is a tried and true wives' tale that adding lemon juice to your water and consuming it first thing upon waking is one of the best treats you can give to your entire body, especially your gut. Many say that drinking it warm is also a key factor for optimal health. Personally, this gave me nausea, albeit mild nausea, but a queasy stomach nonetheless. But it is said to be good for you, so see what your body thinks.

One final surefire way to succeed in hydrating enough throughout the day is to simply focus on drinking 8 ounces of something each hour. For those who spend a fair amount of time at a desk of sorts, this should be a fairly easy habit to get into. Just track every hour on the hour and make sure the 8 ounces is gone by the next o'clock!

YOUR ~~FISCAL~~ PHYSICAL RETIREMENT PLAN

By paying attention to your hydration levels, you keep your body stable with hydration and homeostasis. We lose water through urination, sweat, talking and breathing. If you are doing any of these in excess (and we know you do that last one at least 20,000 times a day), drink your water! The more respect you give to how your body is feeling with hydration levels, the more stable and balanced it is, allowing it to focus on other priorities!

WHERE YOU SHOULD SPEND 1/3 OF YOUR LIFE: ASLEEP!

It seems this is how humans are designed. We are meant to be awake for 16 hours a day and at rest for 8. Within those 8 hours, dozens of biological processes go on that help us to wake up and function every day. Our bodies need that time to complete those processes. However, most of us don't get enough sleep to accomplish all that the body needs to! According to the Centers for Disease Control, one third of Americans are getting less than 7 hours of sleep per night.

If you remember in the *I. A.M. H.E.R.E.* chapter, there are a multitude of things that can contribute to illness and poor brain function, and sleep plays a major role. (Please review that chapter again – under the "R" for Rest – it is important.) Sleep should be a priority in your life. In order to help you recognize the need for more sleep and also find a way to do that, here is a plan to help you get into an 8-hour sleep cycle:

As a starting point, let's assume you are getting 6 hours of sleep and need to add 2 hours per night. I know, this may sound really easy, but for many it is not. It might be easy to get into bed early to try to gain an hour, but sleep deprivation also can be due to stress and a mind that will not stop. If you get up at 6:00am, then you should be asleep at or before 10:00pm, which means lights out around 9:45pm.

Decide which end of the day is more flexible to get that extra hour or two, or you can split the time and add extra sleep time at each end of the day. Now, to start, rather than trying to add that hour all at once, just add five minutes. Simply go to bed five minutes earlier and do that for one week. So, if you have been in bed with lights out at 11:00pm, have lights out at 10:55pm. Adjust your timing based on the time you need to get up in the morning.

Each week add another 5 minutes. In this example, using 5-minute time changes, you will be able to get your 8 hours each night after 3½ months. Though you might think that is a long time, it is not, considering it is for the rest of your life.

There is a reason that the intervals are only 5 minutes: Your body will not recognize the transition and will be more compliant. If, all of a sudden, you went to bed an hour earlier, it is possible that you will just lie there and fall asleep an hour later. But, a 5-minute difference will most likely go unnoticed.

The exception is for those of you who wake up fully rested, naturally (no alarm clock needed) and are not tired at all. You are ready to burst forth into the day and have only gotten seven hours of sleep. Please consider yourself lucky! You're getting an appropriate amount of sleep for YOU, and you get an extra hour of wakefulness each day!

A Quick Word About Your Circadian Rhythm

Our Circadian Rhythm is the rhythm that our body acquires in concert with its own systems as well as the earth and its rotations and daily cycles. For instance, when the outside begins to go dark as night falls, melatonin is enhanced and cortisol is reduced to help tell us that it is time to get tired and go to bed. In the morning, when the sun comes up and we sleep in an undarkened room, our body switches the prominent hormone to wake us up – melatonin is reduced as cortisol is increased. When we sleep in rhythm with darkness and light, we are sleeping in the natural rhythms of the planet. Some say this is the healthiest way to sleep. Granted, as the seasons change, there are far fewer hours in the day during the winter and it is not realistic to sleep for the number of dark hours that there are.

I would say, though, if you are that seven-hours-a-night sleeper, you might want to try the extra hour of sleep and see how your body responds. You might be surprised! Even though you think seven hours is enough, you could be wrong. Your future health is very dependent on all your body's systems functioning properly and in balance. A full night's sleep is one of the most important ways to support those systems to function to the best of their abilities.

MEDITATION: A CRITICAL "PEACE" OF YOUR AGING JOURNEY

Meditation is one of the hardest practices I have ever tried. There is something about sitting still for 20 minutes that does not equate with my personality. I am an on-the-go person. Always have been and, God willing, always will be. I have a need to feel like I am *doing* something. When meditating, I don't feel like I am doing anything. I know now that I am giving a remarkable gift to my body and mind. However, I carry from childhood a message I got from watching my mom who was constantly "doing."

I knew it was time to seriously adopt meditation to help appease my rising stress levels. And when I checked in with my body and my gut, the resounding answer was yes, this is going to be good. So, the challenge was on! I studied it a bit and chose to incorporate it into my regular early morning routine. As previously mentioned, I adhere to a daily morning practice within a few minutes of waking. When I first started with morning meditations, I started using mala beads.

What are mala beads, you ask? Mala beads are a single string of 108 beads (a magic number!), separated into two sets of 54. You choose a mantra and say it with thumb and forefinger touching a bead, then you move onto the next bead and repeat it - a full 54 times. You then switch hands and do the same thing for the next 54 beads, finishing your 108 Mala Bead Chant.

> ## 108 MALA BEADS
>
> There are many explanations for the number 108. This is my favorite, but please explore, because you never know – you might find something you like better.
>
> - Human beings have 6 senses: Sound, Sight, Smell, Taste, Touch and Consciousness.
> - With the senses, there are 3 possible emotions that can emerge as reactions to sense stimulation - Positive, Negative or Neutral.
> - If you multiply the 6 Senses by the 3 reactions, you get 18 feelings.
> - Each of those 18 emotional reactions have two possible results: pleasure or displeasure.
> - When you multiply 18 by 2 you get 36.
> - These are called the 36 passions.
> - They each have the potential of 3 manifestations: Past, Present or Future.
> - 36 x 3 = 108. 108 possibilities for manifestation.

When I started this form of meditation, my atrial fibrillation was really bad, so the mantra I chose to repeat was, "My heart is healthy, my heart is strong, my heart is healed" for each bead. As the AFib subsided, I chose to use Sanskrit words and other mantras. Now, I pause to create one small thought that is inspiration for my entire day and I repeat that. The important part when using mala beads is to sit focused on one thing – and make that the meditation.

Once my morning routine was down pat, I gradually started to add an afternoon walk every day – I am blessed that I live about a half mile from the ocean. I have found a giant rock that I call my own and that is where I stop, sit and just watch the water. I breathe slowly, focus on just my breath and let the sound of the waves create a natural rhythm. The length of time varies, sometimes ten minutes, other times maybe twenty. I know I have a spectacular view and I am grateful for that, but it really isn't important that you have a special view. What is important is that you find a space outdoors if at all possible. Getting in touch with the harmony found in all nature helps your body to assimilate harmony within itself. Even better is to go barefoot and allow the energy of the earth to flow into the energy of your body. When you become one with nature, your body's energy will synchronize and be synergized in this connection. And breathe. Simply breathe and focus on your breathing. This is something I wish I had learned so much longer ago!

A Plan to Get Started

When you first begin to meditate, simply see how long you can sit comfortably without getting distracted. As soon as you are distracted, make note of how long you were able to sit. That is your baseline. Work with that baseline and each week, add 30 seconds – then 60 seconds. In six months you can work up to 20 minutes a day of calm meditative time. And from there, you have the rest of your life to keep it up!

Remember I shared that there are all kinds of meditation? Maybe you want to try just being mindful of the nature surrounding you. It is still important to sit and focus on your breath – it is always about the breath. Be present in the current moment and simply note and appreciate all that surrounds you - the grass, the bushes, the butterfly, the flies, the backyard, the leaves, the weeds! Any and all animals, the rocks, the gravel – it does not matter! What matters is there are no outside thoughts coming in. You are simply taking things in and accepting … and breathing. If you are a high-energy type like me, you really should start to incorporate this into your life – it is a practice that only offers good things for you.

There is another place you can be mindful - that is while driving! We are so used to driving with distractions, whether it's the GPS, the radio, listening to podcasts, and whatever it is that filters in while we drive. But imagine just driving and being present to all that is around you - the scenery, the other cars, the road, the billboards. Try to drive in silence and focus on what is your "now" … and breathe. If another thought comes into your brain, acknowledge it, be grateful for it, then move on and get back to driving. I do this quite frequently when I need to relax and "chill out." It is an amazing way to unwind and also a much safer way to drive! And, when you find yourself stuck behind that driver that is moving at a turtle's pace, maybe it is really the Universe's way of telling *you* to slow down!!

HOW TO INCORPORATE EXERCISE INTO YOUR LIFE

An Hour A Day Keeps The Doctor Away!

Believe me, I can hear your reaction: "An *hour* a day?? I don't have that kind of time!"

Of course you don't – at least not right now. But you can and you will!

This all has to do with making health a priority as you schedule your day. There are a million reasons NOT to take an hour a day to exercise your body and only one reason why you should: exercise is the heart and soul of your health.

Exercise is the one form of activity whose sole purpose is for the betterment of your overall health and wellness. If your day is the typical 16-hour day, we are only talking 1/16th (or 6%) of that! How can you NOT give back to yourself for just an hour a day?

You need to find exercise that you enjoy doing and is in fact, exercise. As discussed in *Exercise Is A Gift*, sports and routine activities do not count. What counts is that the hour is dedicated to your body, mind and spirit. You do not want any outside influences or distractions, such as winning a game!

Some suggestions for you are walking, bike riding, aerobics, step aerobics, Zumba, water aerobics, Pilates, kickboxing, swimming, dancing, stair climbing, hiking, rock climbing, spin classes...the list is endless!

Look for cardio exercises you could do several days a week and start there. Did you know long walks are acceptable? One of my favorite choices is a three-mile morning walk. Another morning I might opt for step aerobics, then a yoga class on Saturdays and a 4-mile hike on the weekends. Another schedule I have done successfully is to do a 2-to-3-mile walk each morning

YOUR ~~FISCAL~~ PHYSICAL RETIREMENT PLAN

followed by 20 minutes of strength training. Right now, I strength train and stretch for 45 minutes in the morning and walk for 45-60 minutes after dinner. Needless to say, the "after dinner" needs to be adjusted in the winter hours, but I do the walking later in the day.

Your schedule will be what works best for you, both in the exercise you choose and the time you have to do it. So don't be discouraged if the first way you organize your schedule of exercises doesn't really work for you. Just try something else.

You want to balance out the body's demands and make sure that there are two days between strength training exercises of the same muscle groups. Take another look at the *Exercise Is A Gift* chapter for some ways to vary the exercises you choose. But if you are just starting out, establishing a discipline is the most important challenge at hand. There are many different approaches you can take. Over the years I have had the most success with clients starting right away with 5 days a week: Monday-Friday, or whatever days are your "work week." That way you begin immediately to incorporate this new way of life on a daily basis when your time is most organized and precious.

When starting, however, I certainly do not recommend an hour a day. At the beginning, the time allotment is more about getting it on your calendar and fulfilling the commitment. It's not so much about the exercise, it's about showing up. As long as you maintain the commitment, you are further along than you were before you started.

The following is a breakdown of how you can actually ease into the regimen of exercising 5 days a week building to one hour a day.

Week One:	10 Minutes each day
Week Two:	20 Minutes each day
Week Three:	30 Minutes each day
Week Four:	40 Minutes each day
Week Five:	50 Minutes each day
Week Six:	60 Minutes each day

If you can progress faster than that, by all means, do so. If you are a part of the Studio BodSpir® Membership, on your strength training days, simply stop your video when the time is up and wait until your next strength training day to continue it.

Remember, always make sure that the last thing you do is stretch! By Week Three, you can follow the 6 Day suggested schedule in the BodSpir® Membership program. By Week Six, you will be right in sync with the one-hour BodSpir® workout. Or, by Week Six, do the half-hour version of the BodSpir® workout and another half-hour of cardio, or take a walk. Building up to an hour each day for exercise is not so much about the training, it's more about the discipline of doing it.

One of the main advantages to *slowly* growing into the process of incorporating exercise into your life on a regular basis is that you probably will not have any aches or pain or soreness from exercising. One of the top reasons why beginners, or even seasoned exercisers, quit is pain or injury. By starting out slowly and gradually, your body can get used to the exercise and be better prepared to perform for you in a healthy and safe way.

Strength Training – The Most Important Form of Exercise

It makes sense, doesn't it? You are strengthening your muscles so that they are stronger and better prepared to accommodate whatever demands you put on them, either through other forms of exercise or just through living each day. Unfortunately, logic does not always succeed in driving us to do the right thing. Throughout the twenty-plus years of teaching strength training (and stretching), I knew this to be truth, however, it has not been an easy "sell," because most people do not want to do it! They know they should, but let's face it, it's time-consuming and boring!! I have discovered however, that it is, in fact, the *most* effective and efficient way to build muscle tissue and to maintain it.

There are many exercise programs claiming bragging rights for being the ones that can make you stronger. I am sure your local gym or senior center has several offerings.

But remember my story about losing 22% of my strength after a month of doing only Pilates and yoga!

Conclusion: Do your entire body with strength training (with respective stretching) twice a week, or break it down as the BodSpir® Membership plan shows. After that, do whatever else you would like to do, Pilates and yoga included. But working with weights is the #1 exercise program that you should incorporate into your weekly schedule, without fail. After that, do whatever is of interest that will work your heart and your muscles. A strength training program (such as BodSpir®) supports everything else you do.

DETOXIFICATION – THE FINAL STAGE OF YOUR PHYSICAL RETIREMENT PLAN

Detoxification is a way to cleanse your body of toxic elements that may have been ingested or breathed or soaked in through your skin. Some toxin intake is inevitable, and it's wise to find a way to get rid of it!

There are many different detox programs available to you. Most detox programs are promoting a beverage concoction to be consumed over a period of time, or a food product that you are required to take while eating. And of course, there is always the fasting approach. While many of these programs can help you on your journey to a healthier you, the majority of them leave you feeling hungry, tired, weak, and sometimes nauseous. And if you start a detox program while your diet consists of mostly unhealthy foods, you will most likely feel sick and nauseous for days in your attempt to eliminate all the bad food at once. That is literally your body detoxing.

How Should One Detox?

The most comfortable way to detox is to rid your body of the bad food that was causing much of your toxicity in the first place. In other words, start by changing your diet as you have read previously, especially eating organic as much as possible. If you still wish to detox you can do that when all the bad foods are gone and your body is relatively free of pesticides and food toxins. You will probably notice improvement in your energy levels, how you sleep and generally how you feel all over! At this level of health, the next stage is to incorporate intermittent fasting into your day.

Intermittent Food Fasting

There are as many books about fasting as there are ways to fast. What I can share with you is that it has been well documented that controlled fasting – going without food – is a healthy way to energize your body and maintain healthy functioning of all your systems.

It is critical that you approach fasting carefully and with full attention to the signals your body gives you as you are in the process of fasting. I highly recommend you do this slowly. Rather than a full 24 hours, start by reducing your food intake to a 10-hour window – meaning you will only eat between the hours of 9:00am and 7:00pm, for example. Other than that, you will only drink water - perhaps with lemon. You know you should drink water throughout your day but it is critical you do this when you are fasting!

If that period of eating time is too small, start with a 12-hour window then slowly reduce it. But if you can, try that schedule for a few days in a row. It is a great way for the body to focus on functioning without the distraction of digestion. When this amount of time gets comfortable, reduce it by another hour. When that gets comfortable, reduce it by another hour again.

This is Daily Intermittent Fasting and has become quite popular because it is purported be very healthy. I currently only eat between 10:00am and 6:00pm each day. That is what works best for both my schedule and my body.

Once your body is accustomed to intermittent fasting, you may want to try a full-day fast. With my eating schedule as an example, that would mean not eating from Friday 6:00pm until Saturday at 6:00pm. When doing a fast of this length for the first time, you want to stay close to home, keeping

YOUR ~~FISCAL~~ PHYSICAL RETIREMENT PLAN

yourself in a safe environment and remembering to continuously hydrate. You could get lightheaded or feel out of sorts. Be sure to discuss this with your doctor.[77] You can then determine when or how long you want to fast in the future. Please do your research and make sure that what you choose is not only good for you, but that someone close to you knows what you are undertaking. Always better to be safe than sorry.

Once you and your body get more familiar with fasting, you might want to try what many do: at the beginning of each season, do a 24-48-72-hour fast. Kind of like a seasonal cleanse. Again, if you decide to do this, be sure you have supervision, and do your research to make sure you are being as safe and cautious as possible for your body's sake.

Heavy Metal Detoxification

Have you heard of heavy metals in the body? This is another form of toxicity – heavy metals that have invaded our bodies, particularly mercury.

Many of us have dental cavities that have been filled with mercury fillings. Should you decide to have these removed and replaced with a non-toxic filling, the procedure would have to be done by a biological dentist. Beyond the toxic fillings, our mouths are teeming with bacteria. A biological dentist understands the relationship between our mouths and our overall health and can assist you in cleaning out the toxins that dwell there.

Our exposure to toxins goes beyond mercury fillings. "Every day, we are exposed to thousands of toxic chemicals through products like pharmaceuticals, pesticides, packaged foods, household products, and environmental pollution. Exposure happens simply with our air, food and water. As we have become more accustomed to consuming chemical-laden products, and as our environment has become more contaminated, we have been confronted with an accelerating rate of chronic illnesses like cancer, heart disease, chronic fatigue syndrome, chemical sensitivity, autism

---

[77] Check out some of the resources included in the *You Are What You Eat* Chapter. Many of them have write-ups on fasting.

spectrum disorders, ADD/ADHD, autoimmune disorders, Parkinson's disease, and Alzheimer's disease."[78]

"In a study spearheaded by the Environmental Working Group (EWG) in collaboration with Commonweal, researchers at two major laboratories found an average of 200 industrial chemicals and pollutants in umbilical cord blood from 10 babies born in August and September of 2004 in U.S. hospitals. Tests revealed a total of 287 chemicals in the group. The umbilical cord blood of these 10 children, collected by Red Cross after the cord was cut, harbored pesticides, consumer product ingredients, and wastes from burning coal, gasoline, and garbage.... Of the 287 chemicals we detected in umbilical cord blood, we know that 180 cause cancer in humans or animals, 217 are toxic to the brain and nervous system, and 208 cause birth defects or abnormal development in animal tests."[79] This is the *blood from the umbilical cords of newborn babies*. How do their tiny new bodies deal with all this poison?

I am not trying to scare you, but you have to know, our bodies are full of these toxins! There are tests available to discern what toxins you might have, and ways to get rid of them, if you should decide to explore detoxifying from these pollutants. It is a question of how much you would like to do and how much you are willing to spend. (Two resources for further research are blumhealthmd.com and myersdetox.com.)

You can also invest in a water filtration system to purify your water, and an air filtration system to purify your air at home. The easiest thing you can do is to switch your cleaning products to safer non-toxic ones. You can also eliminate consumption of toxins from your hair and skin care products, including makeup. If you are using any with toxic ingredients, as they are being absorbed into your skin they are also being absorbed into your bloodstream. (I read something a few years ago that stated the average woman who wears makeup everyday ends up absorbing over 2 pounds of

---

[78] myersdetox.com, "The Shocking Amounts of Toxic Chemicals in Your Body"
[79] ewg.org (Environmental Working Group), "Body Burden: The Pollution in Newborns," July 14, 2005

YOUR ~~FISCAL~~ PHYSICAL RETIREMENT PLAN

makeup a year. You really want to make sure you know what ingredients are in that makeup!)

Let's go back to the beginning and restate our biggest goal – to help the body maintain homeostasis and balance! The less effort your body has to spend on internally detoxing your body from all the poisons, the more energy it has to give you health and vitality and deter the development of chronic disease. That is why all of this gets a mention.

So, to eliminate toxins from your life, go through your home cleaning products, and one by one, finish the bottle that you are on and when replacing it, find a product that is cleaner than the one you are using. Same goes for your skin and hair care products. Everything that touches my body – cleanser and toner, shampoo and conditioner, moisturizer and makeup – is organic. It took some time to find the brands that work for me, but there is plenty of available information online. One by one, as they ran out, I replaced with an organic brand. It took well over a year to replace everything, but I was able to find organic replacements for every product I use.

YOUR PHYSICAL RETIREMENT PLAN

Regardless of your fiscal situation, your physical retirement plan can begin NOW! By educating yourself and making better choices, you are supporting a healthy lifestyle that will see you well into your nineties.

Remember to use baby steps with everything to help set yourself up for success. If you choose to do the 1-10 scale with every behavior because it worked with your food choices, by all means do. Whatever it takes to move you closer to your success.

As with most challenges or changes, the more effort you put in, the more benefit you will receive. While this is ultimately your choice, it is my hope you will see the benefits of controlling your physical future and do what needs to be done now. As passionate as I am about this for you, it is equally upsetting when I see someone needlessly falling victim to ill health. You want to be that vibrant contributor to your family and your community, not a burden to them.

One last thing about implementing your Physical Retirement Plan: Be kind to yourself as you implement these changes in your life. Flexibility with your "rules" might mean that your progress takes longer, but your success will be met with pride and self-assuredness. Focus on what you can do and make it better. We need to re-program our brains, in a sense. Typically, we go to what is wrong and fix it, rather than what we do right and enhance it. Look at everything as a strength, just some needing more effort than others. Recognize how you enhance the strengths you already have and use that talent to help your lesser strengths get stronger.

The more you incorporate the behavior changes into your daily and/or weekly routine, the more likely you are to be successful.

CHAPTER 13 RECAP

1) When thinking of retirement, every one of us needs to give equal consideration to our health AND to our finances.
2) What if there were a plan to change your behavior that was progressive in nature but not massively transitional from the start, where there were a checks-and-balances system so that you are always moving towards the ultimate goal? What if the plan were designed to inspire and encourage you with a realistic approach? What if the plan were unique to you: customized for your specific dreams and desires, your specific capabilities and your specific dietary needs? And, what if you had twenty years to complete it?
3) Whether it is dealing with climate change or knowing that we absolutely need to change our diet and eliminate certain foods, we are a reactionary society, not a proactive one. Consequently, we typically need some sort of catalyst in our face to get us to do something when changing our behavior.
4) The easiest way to be successful when changing behavior is to use baby steps. Don't try to do every change all at once. Break it down and do

YOUR ~~FISCAL~~ PHYSICAL RETIREMENT PLAN

the least amount of change, see how easy it was, then slowly increase the kind of change you are making. This way you are constantly succeeding, albeit with baby steps, but who cares, as long as it is in the right direction.

5) Having a hard time giving up sugar? Studies with rats have proven that sugar is 8 times more difficult to give up than cocaine!

6) The bottom line for optimal health is knowing that most disease is caused by inflammation. Most inflammation is caused by stress, toxins and food. Because food choices and how we oversee our stress are completely under our control, we can change, manage, and eliminate inflammation and most toxins.

7) To help you eliminate the "bad" foods from your diet, there is a systematic approach which breaks things down into much smaller groups of foods to be eliminated. Your chances for success are better if you spread it out over time and just do a small number of foods, even just one food, that you eliminate at a time.

8) When creating your retirement plan for hydration, you want to make sure that you drink enough water and fluid each day to maintain homeostasis. If you need to build to this, that can be done in a gradual approach that will not shock your body or your kidneys.

9) We are meant to be awake for 16 hours a day and at rest for 8. Within those 8 hours, dozens of biological processes go on that help us to wake up and function every day. Our bodies need that time to complete those processes. However, most of us don't get enough sleep to accomplish all that the body needs to!

10) Practicing meditation is one of the greatest gifts you can give to your body. There are lots of different ways to meditate and you need to try as many as you wish until you find what works for you. Start out slowly and gradually build to 20 minutes, maybe even twice a day, but allow yourself as much as a year to get there…baby steps!

11) Exercise is the one form of activity whose sole purpose is the betterment of your overall health and wellness. If your day is the typical 16-hour day, we are only talking $1/16^{th}$ (or 6%) of that! How can you NOT give back to yourself for just an hour a day?

12) Working with weights is the #1 exercise program that you should incorporate into your weekly schedule without fail. After that, do

whatever is of interest that will work your heart and your muscles. A strength training program (such as BodSpir®) supports everything else you do.

13) Detoxification is a way to cleanse your body of toxic elements that may have been ingested or breathed or soaked in through your skin. Some toxin intake is inevitable, and it's wise to find a way to get rid of it!

14) There are several ways to detox and it makes sense to do your research to find the one that is right for you. Keep in mind, some detoxification programs can make you feel very sick and you should only do them with a doctor's or professional's help.

15) Controlled fasting – going without food for a limited time – is a healthy way to energize your body and maintain healthy functioning of all your systems.

16) Heavy metal toxicity is prevalent everywhere and in everyone. It is important to know the risks for disease it creates in our bodies. There are ways to control what we put in our mouths, on our skins, in our hair and on our nails. We can also control what we clean with in our homes, what we spray in our gardens and on our lawns. It is critical that we take control where we can, which helps give our bodies a fighting chance.

17) Regardless of your fiscal situation, your physical retirement plan can begin NOW! By educating yourself and making better choices, you are supporting a healthy lifestyle that can see you well into your nineties.

18) As with most challenges or changes, the more effort you put in, the more benefit you will receive. While this is ultimately your choice, it is my hope you will see the benefits of controlling your physical future and do what needs to be done now.

19) Be kind to yourself as you implement your Physical Retirement Plan in your life. Focus on what you can do and make it better, one step at a time.

Chapter 14

MOBILITY FOR LIFE: EMOTIONS, ATTITUDES, AND THE ULTIMATE GIFT

"Real change, enduring change, happens one step at a time."
Ruth Bader Ginsburg

Change takes time. Throughout this process of taking control of your aging, it is important that you be your own best cheerleader. Many of the people in your life might not be able to support you in the way you hope or want them to. You need to make sure that *your* inspiration is well intact and that *your* emotions are invested in *your* future health.

EMOTIONS

We are motivated to change based on how we feel. So, get emotional about your "why." Embrace the hard work this will take and the challenges it presents. In the long run, you will rise up as your own superhero and be able to face your longevity with confidence and strength, freedom and independence.

Be kind to yourself with these plans and all the changes you are making in your life. When we approach something with hard and fast rules that have no flexibility, it can lead to resentment, frustration and failure. Being too steadfast to the rules can result in stumbling blocks to your progress. More flexibility provides a surer pathway to success – even if it takes longer than you would like. This is *your* journey - make sure you continue on your path, always heading in the right direction.

Recognize the impact that emotions have on our physical self. As suggested, there is a direct link between emotions and the health of the body. Symptoms or diseases that happen in the body are often the body's way of getting your attention. Just make sure that when your body is trying to speak to you and you decide to listen, you consider both physical and emotional triggers as the possible point of origin.

YOUR ATTITUDE DRIVES YOUR SUCCESS

Your goal is to take control of your physical future, regardless of how long you live. You want to stay focused and stay active. You want to be social and befriend those people who are on a similar path – maybe even share yours and inspire others to join you! Unfortunately, you may discover along the way that some friends are not supportive of your journey, for whatever reason. They could, in fact, be jealous of your conviction.

Remember, it is totally up to you with whom you choose to spend your time.

Loving what you do and doing what you love is definitely in order here. By now, hopefully, you have discovered what thrills you each day. What gets you out of bed in the morning and keeps a smile on your face all day, or at least most of it. Feeling happy is your inner being whispering that you are on the right path … that what you are doing is working … that how you are living is how you are meant to live. When you feel sad or angry or frustrated, it is the opposite message – what you are doing is not jibing with what you are meant to be doing. So stop that behavior and get back on track with what makes you feel good. Your success will only come when you are in the right frame of mind. And, with whatever changes you need to make to your lifestyle to be successful in controlling your aging, you will need to have an upbeat, positive attitude for it all to work.

As you have read in *The Mind-Body Partnership*, your body is always communicating with you. Your true self, your soul, your passion, your purpose – those parts of you that are intrinsically, uniquely YOU – are communicating to you through your heart and feelings and emotions. While your emotions can be complex, they will generally affect you in one of two ways: you feel good or you feel bad. When you feel good, your heart is happy and you are synchronized with your true self. When you feel sad, whatever you are doing or whatever is happening is not synchronized with your true self and you need to change directions. So, as you are learning to listen to your body, remember to respect the emotional communication your body is sending you. And follow your happy!!

Stay positive as often as you can. If something is making you feel yucky inside, try to look at it from the opposite perspective. How could the same thing that makes you feel miserable help to make you feel joyful? Your perspective is what matters. For example, say you were looking forward to doing some gardening when the skies open up and it is clearly going to rain all day. What indoor project would give you a real sense of accomplishment? Or the in-laws are coming for Thanksgiving and it is always a nightmare. What new recipes and dishes could you prepare this year to distract you from the negativity? Keeping a positive spin on the negative situations not only makes them more fun and tolerable, but often helps you accomplish new things you would not necessarily have attempted.

The bottom line to your success in this venture will have everything to do with what you think about rather than what you do. How you think will actually play a giant role in determining the outcome. If you think it will be difficult to change your diet, it will be. If you think exercise is a hard discipline to attain, it will be. If you think eighty is old, then it is. If you expect some chronic disease will overthrow your life by the time you are 75, it will. Your future wellbeing depends on your actions, but it also depends very heavily on how you think.

How you think is mostly derived from your childhood experiences, experts say, between birth and age 6 or 8, and how you have interpreted those thoughts determines your attitudes as an adult. This isn't just how you think about other things, it is also how you think about yourself. The choices you make in life are determined by your attitudes about you in relationship to your life and its challenges and opportunities. Your success in achieving every new behavior will depend entirely on your attitude about it.

I repeat that great Henry Ford quote, "If you think you can do a thing or think you can't do a thing, you're right."

Owning a positive and grateful attitude every step of the way will guide you to a successful outcome, met with glory and self-assuredness. Being positive and connecting with your heart for all decisions will make it easier to embrace the discipline needed to move forward.

Never forget: You are completely in charge of how you live the rest of your life.

THE ULTIMATE GIFT

There is one thing that I have barely mentioned throughout this book and it is the backbone of everything written here. Make no mistake, the discipline you need to change destructive behaviors is extremely challenging. You will never be perfect at it, so don't expect to be. But the tasks at hand will be much easier to address if you have this one thing. These challenges will never appear as obstacles, only opportunities -- some more perplexing and difficult than others, but all very doable.

That one gift you need to give yourself every step of the way is **SELF-LOVE**. And, ultimately, do you love yourself enough to do the right thing and make the right choice?

MOBILITY FOR LIFE: EMOTIONS, ATTITUDES, AND THE ULTIMATE GIFT

From *The Mind-Body Partnership* chapter when speaking about Lucille: *What it really comes down to is self-love. Did I love myself enough to finally be kind, considerate and loving to <u>me</u>? Did I love myself enough to NOT feed myself those foods that would do harm to my body? After all, if Lucille were my constant companion, so was I!*

Are you blessed to have self-love already? I certainly wasn't.

Sharing My Story

Please understand, it's not that I was not loved as a child. I certainly was. It was my *interpretation* of my parents' behavior towards me that created the attitudes I had. But my journey is solely mine to travel, and I had a need to learn self-love.

As a matter of fact, it wasn't until I reached my sixties that I was able to truly grasp and embrace the concept. Here is what happened.

One day I posted a general inquiry on Linked In. I was seeking information about research that I hoped had been done connecting the use of pesticides with the rise in disease. (A passion of mine, as you have learned.)

I was connected with an "Emotional Energy Healer" in western Canada – about as far away in North America as you can get from me. He could not answer my research questions, but he did have this amazing emotional healing expertise. Honestly, I wasn't even aware I needed this, but when we remain openminded, we quickly learn that the Universe always knows more than we do!

With his guidance, over a series of weekly sessions, I looked back at my childhood. I realized that my mother was not crazy about babies, so I never really got held much or played with as a baby. I know I spent countless hours in a playpen, by myself. When my dad got home from work, they had a routine: It was time for cocktails. This was my mom's way of supporting him. How did Dad interact with me? Maybe I got a pat on the cheek or a tease, but that was the extent of his ability to interact. They did the best they could, based on how they were taught!

Fast forward to my school years and off my mom went to work. Back then, that was a rarity. She was among the very few "working moms" in our neighborhood. I would go to a neighbor's house after school until I was around age 10, when I became a latchkey kid. Roll the life film reel forward. As I grew, I began to participate in after-school sports. There was not one single game that either parent ever attended. It was never discussed why they didn't or couldn't attend. This went on through high school; I was always active on a sports team or involved in school activities that other parents attended. My parents' absence and lack of support in my life had a profound effect on me that I didn't understand at the time.

Again, I had a nice home and was well provided for and wanted for nothing. I knew in my head that I was loved, but I wanted to know it in my heart. Who knew that it would take almost sixty years for me to overcome the lack of a sense of self-worth that had developed those many, many years ago?

With this emotional healer's help, I was able to go back to my childhood and look at all the reasons why I "believed" I was unlovable and unworthy. With his guidance and suggestions, I was able to get through the pain of discovery and awareness and let go of the scared little girl whose defense mechanisms had protected her all these years. At last I could embrace the new-found adult woman with whom I face every new day.

The Universe continued its expansion, guiding me to all sorts of self-healing podcasts, websites and experts as well as showing me online courses I could take.

Once I accepted and grew to love myself, my fitness journey became so much easier and so much more enjoyable! I no longer wanted to "cheat" with unhealthy foods because I didn't want to poison myself – why would I poison someone I loved so much?

I am no longer vulnerable, and any kind of victimhood has been obliterated. I am free to love myself and have grown strong and confident, accepting all my qualities – whether others do or not – I am not here to "please" them. I have trust and confidence in the guidance I receive from my heart and have an incredibly strong understanding that I am on the right path with all that I do. If not, there is always a sign cluing me in to take another look. I am very much at peace and am blessed to love myself, warts and all, as the saying goes!

Before this revelation, I worked my program because I should. After learning self-love, I did it because I wanted to. I stepped out of the world of *self-harm* (knowingly eating nonorganic/toxic foods, for example) into the world of self-love. I became much more disciplined with all the regimens discussed in the *I. A.M. H.E.R.E.* chapter because I knew how good it was for me and I was worthy of feeling healthy and fit.

No matter what stage of growth you have achieved or what disciplines you have grasped, you will find that **putting yourself first and making the best decisions for you and embracing those decisions are the purest form of self-love there is**. And everything you do for *you* automatically enriches those around you who love you.

Sharing Lulu's Story

If you have seen the possibilities and have done the activities and plans that are suggested in this book (including "Discovering Your Aha!"), but you still find it difficult to apply the discipline needed, could it be that deep down you are still not feeling worthy to attain healthy living for decades to come?

I know it might sound like a bit of a stretch, but in all the years I have been doing this work with clients, I look back and realize that it is the feeling of unworthiness that is behind more failure in meeting personal dreams and desires than any other reason.

I want to share Lulu's story. Lulu is not her real name. She was in her mid-50s and had a wonderful and comfortable life, but her self-care was lacking. She was overweight by about 50 pounds and her mobility was weakening each year. She could have anything money could buy, but she could not buy the discipline she needed to stay on track. She could go months at a time, lose 20 pounds, be diligent with everything, then go away for a month and whoosh! When she returned it was like we had barely done any work and we would have to backtrack, re-group and start all over again. One day we discussed the concept of self-worthiness, or lack thereof.

Eagerly, she ventured back into her childhood and related that when she was four years old, she had to move away from home with some other family members, not able to see or visit her core family. When she was eight years old, she was returned to her original family.

She had never really considered how much of an impact that had on her life.

She was well cared for and loved in both places, but the abandonment of her core family left a huge gap in her need to be loved. If her core family abandoned her, even though they eventually took her back, why was she worthy of self-love? So, we took a look at the ramifications of what had happened and how that innocent child must have interpreted those actions.

Looking back on this period of her life from an adult perspective gave her a huge "Aha!" moment which was just the catalyst she needed. That, along with a couple of other tools to help guide her, gave her the ability to dive into some self-love very quickly. Within eight months those 50 pounds were gone, never to return. She took up bike riding long distances and felt confident and sure she was now in control. She could openly look forward to a life of health and vitality for the next fifty years or more!

Lulu's battle with her weight throughout her life is not unusual for anyone who has suffered or continues to suffer from obesity. Many factors contribute to obesity and more research is being done continuously. The body's metabolism has a strong influence on how you react to weight loss and whether you will regain the weight or keep it off. If you are obese (defined as having a Body Mass Index over 30), I strongly recommend that you seek out an obesity professional who is familiar with both conventional and alternative options to help with the perfect plan for you to gain control over your body.

Our attitude about our weight – our subconscious approach to our weight and our relationship with food – was derived from what we learned in childhood. So, what caused the overeating in the first place? When we can look into our souls and answer that question honestly, a light goes on and our pathway becomes clear!

SOME SIMPLE IDEAS TO GET YOU STARTED

Love the Child You Were

One of the tools I shared with Lulu was one that my energy healer had shared with me.

I found some pictures of myself at different stages of my childhood, ranging from age two to sixteen. I put them in a collage and hung it over my bureau (where it still hangs). On the bottom of the frame, I put a sticky note that reads: "I will love you now." Every day, I look at that little girl/young woman and tell her how much I love her, even if I were unable to love her then.

Say a Simple "I Love You!"

Another wonderful activity to help you down the self-love road is something I learned from the teachings of Louise Hay of Hay House Publishing. Initially this can be a very uncomfortable activity in all its simplicity. It is what she calls her mirror work.

Start with a handheld mirror. Look yourself straight in the eye and say, "I love you. I really, really love you!"

Now, I know this sounds corny and awkward and silly, but *it works!!* If you do this each day at the start of your day, by the end of the first week the awkwardness begins to dissipate and the tears begin to flow -- cleansing tears and tears of joy! You are actually declaring your love for yourself to yourself! What could be more self-affirming than that?

Embrace the Beauty of the Earth

Go out in nature more often – it does wonders for the soul! Walk barefoot on the ground so that you can harmonize with Mother Earth and her magnificent energy that she so graciously and generously synergizes with yours. You deserve it!

Forgive Those You Need to Forgive

I am sure, if you have lived past the age of 40, that there are some people along the way that have done you wrong. Some of them may still be in your life. Fortunately, I do not see the couple who used to be friends that did me wrong by borrowing money and never paying me back – a LOT of money. I have had to forgive them for being such bad people and destroying our friendship. I have had to forgive others who ignored what they did to me, and I have had to forgive myself for trusting them and believing in them.

Forgiveness doesn't really have much to do with them anyway. It has much more to do with you. "Forgiveness is associated with better physical health and predictive of fewer physical health symptoms. Forgiveness leads to healthier cardiovascular responses to stress and lower rates of cardiovascular disease. Forgiveness is linked with less risk of earlier death."[80]

With forgiveness, you recognize that you really don't have any control over other people's behavior. And even though what someone may have done to you is not something you could ever imagine doing to anyone, it doesn't matter. Because their behavior doesn't change who you are and you have no control over their behavior. However, your behavior and attitude change you, and you have total control over that.

So, as you venture forth on this new chapter in your life of self-care and self-love, I suggest you take a look around and see if there are any outstanding grudges you may be holding. Now would be a really good time to let them go. Embrace the new positive-thinking, forward-moving you and forgive those close to you that have hurt you. Then, once forgiven,

---

[80] *IDEAFit*, "The Forgiveness Factor," Lee Jordan, MS, and Beth Jordan, March 3, 2020

you get to choose whether you want to continue to have them in your life or not.

Forgive Yourself

Let's face it, by now in your life you have made some bad choices. We all have. One of the hardest things we have to do as full-fledged adults is to be honest with ourselves about mistakes we have made or hurt we have caused others. Unfortunately, we bury our guilt or shame and don't realize that our regret is eating us up inside.

However, if you can be honest with yourself and *admit* to your mistakes, it will give you a wonderful sense of relief. And to go a step further and actually *forgive* yourself for what you have done, whether it is harm or hurt to another or oneself, that is the biggest freedom of all.

Regret really weighs heavily on us as we get older – not just with the choices we made that were the wrong choices, but the choices we didn't make that would have been the right ones.

Have a journaling session, or two or three. Perhaps enlist the help of a coach or therapist or a trusted friend. Go through your life, decade by decade, and see if there are things that you did or did not do that you still regret. If there is a way to atone for some hurt you have caused others, by all means, do it. But whatever you discover, forgive yourself for making the choice that you made, then let it go. Write it down on a piece of paper, light a match to it and let it go.

Gratitude. Gratitude. Gratitude.

It is an interesting time we are living in when we are all so busy that we have to be reminded to be grateful. I am referring to the massive number of studies and data suggesting that gratitude and the state of being grateful can increase your serotonin, make you happier, relieve stress and generate a multitude of other feel-good emotions. Funny thing is, it's true. Thinking about that for which you are thankful on a daily basis helps you sleep better and puts a smile on your face! At least it did for me when I started doing a brief gratitude journal before bed. And I do mean brief.

I have a monthly calendar with one box for each day and I write at least 3 things for which I am grateful for that day. It is part of my nighttime ritual. And, I have to say, it has helped with my peace of mind and my moods, as well as my sleep.

The "things" I write down are not necessarily big things, either. And there are some things for which I am grateful every day. If I am too lazy to pick up the calendar, I will just lie in bed before I turn the light out and think and feel the gratitude for that day.

It is particularly helpful if I have had a bad day. It's like putting on that pair of rose-colored glasses and having a different viewpoint or perspective. Being grateful also helps if you have just had a horrific experience or phone call or argument. Simply close your eyes, take a few slow, deep breaths (in through the nose and out through the mouth), get centered, focus on that which makes you happy and say thank you. You will be amazed, after just a minute or two, how much better you feel.

Don't Put Off Today...

There is no time like the present. There will never be a perfect time to start. Just start. I remember trying to plan when to have children. I was told countless times that you can never pick the right time because life just doesn't work that way. It is never the perfect time. So, just start.

Another stall tactic is to have one goal depend on another. For instance: Let me lose the weight first, then I will start feeling better about myself. Instead, feel better about yourself today and the weight will come off more easily.

Remember, procrastination has nothing to do with the task and everything to do with your relationship with the task. Your emotions are stirred with what you are setting forth to do, not actually what you are doing. So, if it really is hard to get going with one of your plans, look more at what the plan entails and what part of it causes you to be fearful or unsure. What if there were no fear of failure, but actually a fear of success?

When venturing forth on your wellness journey, you must first reflect on where you are now. Don't dwell on how you got there, but recognize where you are. Do your own body scan and focus on what your body can do, not what it can't. And say thank you with each part, just like we did in the I. A.M. H.E.R.E. meditation. As your journey progresses and you get stronger and more fit, you will find yourself saying thank you to your body a lot!

Write It Down!

When you start out with all your plans as suggested, do make sure you write down your goals with each plan. In baby steps. For some reason, putting pen to paper triggers more of a commitment. It has made the goal more concrete, more real. It is no longer something that you are just thinking about or that you wish would happen. You are actually making it more tangible.

Become the Role Model

What if you took this challenge to control your aging and ran with it? What if you became the motivator to others? What if, as you made more and more progress, you actually became a role model for others who wanted to do what you are doing? The discipline and strength you show with your program is certainly something that others would also want to master. Perhaps even family members who need such focus could be influenced by your behavior. They might even subconsciously help you to set your bar higher for yourself.

Remember what happens when you surpass your goals: Your self-love grows and grows. Your pride in yourself grows. You start to believe in yourself more, and that gets crossed over to other parts of your life with a new confidence and self-esteem. That sense of positive energy flows through you, touching all parts of you, including your brain, nervous system, immune system – all over. Your physical and emotional selves thrive when you are knowingly empowering others.

The most important part of learning self-love is to trust that you are meant to love yourself. You are meant to come first in your own life in order to better serve everyone else. You are meant to make the best choices for your own well-being to not only help yourself but to set an example for others. Unfortunately, this is not something we are taught or encouraged to do as children or as adults. But you know it now and I encourage you to do something with this newfound enlightenment!!

THE FOUR Ds

Another simple approach to changing your lifestyle to one of self-love is found in what I call the 4 Ds: decision, discipline, determination and dedication.[81]

- First of all, you need to make the **decision** that you are going to change the way you take care of yourself. After all, you bought this book!
- Once the decision is made, you will need the **discipline** to follow through with that decision. You've read the specific steps outlined in this book to make the changes. Following those steps will give you the discipline you need.
- A characteristic that will fuel that discipline is your **determination** to become the healthy and fit person you were meant to be. Your determination is supported by the inspiration you found in discovering your "Aha!"
- The 4th and most important D is your **dedication**, not to the program, but to yourself! And you will remain committed to the new you because of the self-love you have discovered!

---

[81] I came up with this on my own, then googled it just in case, and sure enough, there is a book with a pretty close theme: The Four D's Of Life: Desire, Determination, Discipline, Dedication by Cameron Ryan Scott. Also, Brian Tracy discusses it in Eat That Frog.

My brother once told me something about my dad that I was not really conscious of while we were growing up. I think this story perfectly illustrates using the 4 Ds to empower your behavior change in any given moment.

My dad was the epitome of a gentleman. He was always polite and respectful, regardless of the situation. One thing my dad never did was swear! My brother told me that whenever the occasion arose when a good profanity would do the trick, my dad would pause – allowing a split second of sanity – and say something else. It was in that split second that he decided who he was going to be in that moment: He made the **decision** to stop, he had the **discipline** to change his words, he had the **determination** to still express his anger, and he had the **dedication** to maintain his commitment to not swear in front of his children.

Perhaps when you come across a situation in which you are tempted to interrupt your program (for me it was to *not* stop at the ice cream stand!), in that split second, choose who you are going to be: Make the decision not to stop, gather your discipline in not pulling the car into the parking lot, grab onto your determination to envision the healthy person you want to be and say a blessing for the dedication you have to yourself and your lifestyle.

YOUR PATH TO PHYSICAL FREEDOM

It is possible that as you read this, you are not yet aware of your heart's desire and are still on the path of discovering your soul's purpose, your passion. If that is the case, I encourage you to understand how important it is to not let poor health get in the way of your dreams and that you need good health to live the quality of life that your dreams deserve.

If you already know your passion and purpose, then I encourage you to be healthy so you can live it to its fullest.

If you feel fulfilled and you have already lived your heart's desire, how will you live the rest of your life? Will you be in control of your health or will your health be controlling you? The choice is yours.

Being fit and living your life of self-care allows you the freedom to hold onto your hopes and dreams, well into your 90s and beyond. Think about the gift you can give yourself and your family: living a better-than-expected quality of life for extra decades! And, in living longer and healthier, you are partaking in life rather than worrying about becoming a burden to others. You are an active participant in the lives of your family, your friends and your community. Your retirement years could actually be just as long as your working years – imagine all the things you could do if you were in control of your health!

The proven challenges and plans in this book support a life of independence and an ability to live where you want, do what you want, when you want, with whom you choose. You will not need to impose yourself on anyone else because you will be able to take care of yourself. And your quality of life will be exactly what you make of it. You can take full responsibility for all that you do.

There is no one else but you who can do this for you. You are the one who needs to take these steps and make these changes. This is all on you. It is your body. It is your future.

I wish you well on this exciting adventure on which you have chosen to embark. As you succeed, you will be filling up with self-pride and self-love – re-enforcing your path all the more. The rewards are countless and the joy it will bring to you and yours is boundless.

The philosophy is simple:

When you give to your body, your body will respond to you in kind.

The suggestions here take work, time and conditioning, but the rewards are life-long. As much time as it takes to get and stay healthy – whether it's time to work out, extra cooking time, time to meditate, or any other time you need to invest to stay on your path of energetic living – will be minimal when compared to the amount of time that will be taken away due to ill health.

My dream and desire for you is one that has become my life's work. I feel *that passionately* about how I can help:

> ***Giving you the freedom to be physical with your body
> in whatever way you wish, for as long as you wish.***

Remember to love your self and your body, respect your self and your body, and cherish your self and your body.

NAMASTE
Elizabeth Phinney
The Aging Coach

ACKNOWLEDGMENTS

I will start at the beginning with the onslaught of support and encouragement I have received from pretty much everyone I know near and far. What happens when you take almost six years to write a book, pretty much everyone you know learns about it sooner or later. No one ever said, "You haven't finished that yet?" There was only support and encouragement with a whole lot of "attagirls!" Especially from my longest-tenured BodSpir® class attendees. Their loyalty has lasted up to 19 years. Thanks to you guys for always being there and showing up and trusting me to help with your physical stamina all these years.

It was around February of 2018 when I was having dinner with my dear friend, Lavinia. "Phin? Tore (her sister) wants to know why you haven't written your book yet and thought maybe I could be your accountability coach to get you going." Perfect! That is exactly what I needed – someone to whom to be accountable. So, with a great deal of encouragement, Lavinia and I bullied forth to get the outlines done and chapter drafts going. So, to you, dear Verne, I am overwhelmingly grateful for your push and your action on Tore's brilliant idea (Thanks to you, Tore, too!!). Never mind your continued support over the years and your enduring friendship of 55 years and counting!

Once Lavinia and I got going, my very close friend Dianne stepped in. Dianne and I had only known each other for a couple of years at this point, but she had been working with me as a coach for my business and could translate my words into what I really meant to say. So, once I wrote a chapter, I would first send it to Lavinia for the first run through, then on to Dianne for the fine tuning and "translations" to make sure that I got my message across in the best way possible.

More than that, Dianne was becoming my best friend. We had a blast together no matter what we did. She ended up editing almost every chapter and giving back to me a fabulous rendition of many of the words you will read here. The horrible thing is that she never was able to finish my book editing. She died very unexpectedly right before Covid changed all of our lives.

So, to you, my dear, crazy new BFF, I know you are here with me always and will continue with me on this journey. I thank you to the stars and back for all of your love and support.

Losing my coach was certainly not part of the plan. But, as the Universe always provides, within a couple of months, I met a woman via Zoom who was a professional accountability coach. She helps people get things done! And, that is what I needed. Enter Barbara Hubbard from San Diego. Barb and I had weekly calls and goal setting and she helped me with my writing deadlines so I could continue with my focus on the book (as well as the rest of my responsibilities with my mom and managing the house.)

I finally met Barbara in person this past July and after working with her for over a year it was great fun to sit live and in person and chat and laugh and be together. I am incredibly grateful to you, Barb, and your timely entrance into my life. Your calm, articulate manner and graceful friendship has helped keep me on task and focused all the way through the completion of this book. I thank you.

I would also like to thank my dear friend Jessica Martinson who has always believed in me and supported me and graciously encouraged the interruptions that my son would make during our countless conversations.

And, then there is my mom. In the summer of 2008 when I had to find another place to live, I naively asked my 85 year old mother if she thought I should move in. After all, dad was gone and she was getting older. If anything happened to her, I would have to break a lease to move in and help her then. So, why not be prepared? As for me, I figured that she would have company for her last few years and someone to help her as she became more and more aged. Little did I know that it would be 13 years before she would pass.

Mom and I had always had a great friendship and would have great fun together no matter what we did. Living together and care giving presented a completely new set of rules on what defined our relationship.

Somehow, we made it through with our love still intact and her departure has certainly left a hole in my heart. Mom, I want to thank you for ALWAYS supporting me with everything I did, especially this book. And although you will never get to read it, I know you believed in me and always knew I would complete it. I thank you for your faith, your trust and your love.

My acknowledgements would not be complete without mentioning the endless support and love I have always received from my two daughters. We certainly are a trio!! Thank you both to the moon and back for your forever faith and belief in my dreams.

I have saved the best, by far, for last. This book would never have been completed without the help of this woman, and I mean that. When Dianne was still living, I had another friend who would do the edit of the re-edit. I would write, it would go to Dianne. She would edit and send it back to me. I would re-write and send it to Rennie. She would re-edit and send it back to me. And, so it went. Needless to say, when Dianne died, everything kind of halted, for me anyway. But not for Rennie. Within a few months she had compiled the book using all of her editing and presented it to me to read. With all that was going on in my life at the time, especially with my mom, it sat in my inbox for another eight months.

Finally, a year ago January, I pulled it out and we have been back and forth ever since. Rennie, my dear, dear friend of 44 years, how can I ever thank you enough for the countless hours you have spent on perfecting my language and my message? The dedication and stamina that you have shared and your trust in me are humbling, to say the least. Thank you, thank you, thank you, from the bottom of my soul. You epitomize the meaning of friendship and faith. I am forever grateful for your understanding and respect.

ABOUT THE AUTHOR

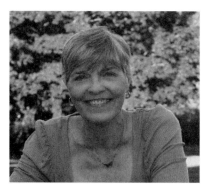

Elizabeth Phinney is a Certified Personal Trainer with the American Council on Exercise. She also holds Specialty Certifications in Fitness Nutrition, Weight Management and Older Adult Fitness. She has been an Affiliate Member of The American College of Sports Medicine for over twenty years.

Elizabeth's passion is to inspire people to create a plan for their physical retirement just as they plan for their fiscal retirement. Over the last 20+ years, she has developed and fine-tuned several fitness techniques and theories that are successfully practiced.

Not only has she spent countless hours helping people get stronger and more flexible, she has helped them slow down, stop, and reverse aging issues that had plagued them for years. In a nutshell, she teaches people how to control how they age, and, just as importantly, that they have that power!

Her flagship product is BodSpir®, a meditative strength training technique she created and has taught thousands of times in her classes and one-on-one private training. Other programs include the F.I.T. Workshop™ (Fitness Inspiration Transformation) and Your Personal C.A.R.E. Package (Consultation, Assessment, Evaluation and Recommendation.) As the Aging Coach™, she helps people prioritize their lifestyle habits so they can give the most back to their bodies as they age.

Visit www.fitnessafterfortyfive.com for further information.